SpringerBriefs in Social Work

More information about this series at http://www.springer.com/series/13578

Emmanuel Janagan Johnson • Camille L. Huggins

Social Casework Methodology: A Skills Handbook for the Caribbean Human Services Worker

Springer

Emmanuel Janagan Johnson
Department of Behavioural
Sciences, St. Augustine Campus
The University of the West Indies
St. Augustine, Trinidad and Tobago

Camille L. Huggins
Department of Behavioural
Sciences, St. Augustine Campus
The University of the West Indies
St. Augustine, Trinidad and Tobago

ISSN 2195-3104 ISSN 2195-3112 (electronic)
SpringerBriefs in Social Work
ISBN 978-3-030-27318-7 ISBN 978-3-030-27319-4 (eBook)
https://doi.org/10.1007/978-3-030-27319-4

This Springer imprint is published by the registered company Springer Nature Switzerland AG
The registered company address is: Gewerbestrasse 11, 6330 Cham, Switzerland

If you've gotten anything at all out of following Christ, if his love has made any difference in your life, if being in a community of the Spirit means anything to you, if you have a heart, if you care— then do me a favour: Agree with each other, love each other, be deep-spirited friends. Don't push your way to the front; don't sweet-talk your way to the top. Put yourself aside, and help others get ahead. Don't be obsessed with getting your own advantage. Forget yourselves long enough to lend a helping hand. **Philippians 2:1-4 (MSG)**

This book is dedicated to my beloved mother
Late Mrs. Suganthi Johnson

Preface

Working in the Caribbean for the past few years, it was striking how different the environment was from other countries and how it altered the prescribed approach when working with clients. Professional practice encircles a diverse range of casework methods including direct work with individuals, families, groups, communities, and policy work on a macro level, to achieve the betterment of all individuals. The International Federation of Social Worker (2001) defines the purpose of professional social work as the promotion of social change, problem-solving in human relationships, and the empowerment and liberation of people to enhance well-being. Those working and advocating for people seek to improve the interaction between people and their social environments by facilitating change on multiple levels, including personal change, change in families, groups, communities, formal institutions, and the societal systems that impact a person in each of these areas. The ability to be equipped with a broad range of knowledge, method, and skills that enable the social service worker to intervene effectively in the various systems in order to influence and impact individuals is essential.

The social casework method has many benefits in providing a solid foundation with a broad range of practice methods. These benefits include a vast yet specific set of skills that enables the social service worker to respond with more flexibility and creatively with clients and communities. A diverse set of skills enables better cooperation among social workers as it enhances our appreciation of the value of different practice approaches offered by agencies and practitioners. For example, with the multiple levels of skills, a social service worker working in an agency can appreciate how the interventions offered by a community level worker may be beneficial to clients entering an agency or a community agency. Similarly, a community worker with knowledge of casework methods is well positioned to identify when a community member may benefit from other kinds of casework or group work interventions. The capacity to articulate the value and practice of a diverse practical yet professional base can also help the social service worker become more polished and professional.

Why the Caribbean? Oftentimes people describe the Caribbean as paradise, with crystal blue waters and specular beaches. So what social problems do these 30 tiny island states have that we must consider as detrimental. What is often overlooked is how complex the Caribbean truly is with residents who have either migrated there voluntarily or were brought to these islands due to slavery or indentureship, hundreds of years ago. There is a history of slavery, emancipation, failed attempts at emancipation, as well as the eradication of indigenous people.

To say the least, the Caribbean has a sordid past with people presently suffering from the remnants of this history. These Caribbean islands have thousands of people who are vulnerable (e.g., poverty, lack of education) and is in need of professional assistance in order to effect social change. Social service workers must be able to speak and understand various languages (e.g., Spanish, English, French, Dutch). They must be culturally humble enough to interact with various cultures and religions (e.g., Hindu, Muslim, Arawak Indians). They must be able to differentiate the definition of various social justice terms in diverse cultures such as Does **equality** mean the same in an indigenous peoples' village as it does in a large city? Does **empowerment** translate in patriarchal homes as opposed to matriarchal focal homes? Lastly, the social service worker must be flexible and build true trust with their clients, where the client is actively participating in the process along with the worker. This is sometimes an untenable task in the Caribbean, where some people lack autonomy due to years of oppressive structural practices.

Social casework method encapsulates diverse and multiple methods that a social service worker must have available, but it does not mean all these methods will be used at the same time. Every social service worker should have some level of specialization in the field and understand a method in order to respond in an increasingly complex practice. Specifically, if you are a social service worker that works in agencies of mental health, child protection, or homeless services. The worker should have a detailed knowledge of matters such as indicators of risk, signs of strength, and evidence of best practices with their specific field. There is also a need for operational specialists in a wide variety of fields of practice. These specialists commit significant proportions of work to develop a deep understanding of the casework method. The term casework method appears simple but it is an intricate set of practices to help the worker attune themselves to the client, build trust, develop a working relationship, set goals, and carry through with interventions.

In this book, there is an introduction of the Caribbean and its diversity of people, the social problems the Caribbean is facing, the current social welfare infrastructure, and how social work education is taught, today. It will then outlay the history of the casework method, as well as the pioneers of the different iterations of this method. The book presents the principles that bracket the casework method as well as the theoretical frameworks that were originally used for the casework method as well as theoretical frameworks needed to work in the Caribbean. The book then journeys the reader through the components of the casework method comprehensively describing the complexity of the client, the worker, the relationship, assessment, and intervention. One of the unique features of the book is that it is a mixture of traditional casework methods with the innovative attributions necessary to work with people in the Caribbean. There is also a workbook component with case studies of people and families situated in the Caribbean along with exercises to improve your problem-solving skills to understand the presenting problems, the assessment, and the intervention for each case. The hope is the material presented in this book deepens the reader's understanding of all the aspects of the casework method and how it is applied in the Caribbean.

St. Augustine, Trinidad and Tobago

Emmanuel Janagan Johnson
Camille L. Huggins

Acknowledgments

There are many people who have been instrumental in the completion of this book and deserving my gratitude. First, I thank the Lord Almighty for the blessings to make this project a success. My sincere gratitude and thanks to my coauthor **Dr. Camille Huggins** who fine-tuned my idea and helped to make this possible. Thanks to my students who over the years have served as the inspiration for the ideas, content, and resources in this book, especially for their contribution in the form of case studies. I thank the Editor, **Jennifer Hadley**; **Sara Yanny-Tillar**, Assistant Editor; and **Sofia Geck**, Editorial Assistant, from Springer, who have been with me throughout this project and who have been diligent in keeping me on track and providing us with excellent feedback. The authors thank the entire editorial team for their tireless work. Special thanks to my Social Work colleagues and other well-wishers who are with me extending their support. Finally, thanks to my academic friends, who were always supportive and committed to helping me see this through.

Very special thanks to my daughter **Jessica Evangelin** and wife **Jane** who sacrificed their time and extended their full support to me to work on this project.

Emmanuel Janagan Johnson

I would like to thank Dr. Emmanuel Janagan Johnson for believing in me enough to collaborate in writing this book. It has been an honor. This would not be possible if it were not for my mother Cynthia Carrington Murray, a single mother who immigrated from Trinidad and Tobago to the United States. She enticed my curiosity and allowed me to pursue my education, as young women of color are often disadvantaged in pursuing their dreams. Part of the impetus for this book is my fifteen years of social work practice in New York City, which provided me with an understanding that students must critically think about appropriate theories in order to properly assess and implement action steps to help our most vulnerable people. The Caribbean is a special place with a diverse and rich history that cannot be ignored when treating clients. The environment in which we live oftentimes determines one's life trajectory. I would also like to thank the University of the West Indies at St. Augustine for the opportunity to work and research in the Caribbean, as it has enriched my life experience.

Camille L. Huggins

Contents

List of Diagrams

List of Tables

About the Authors

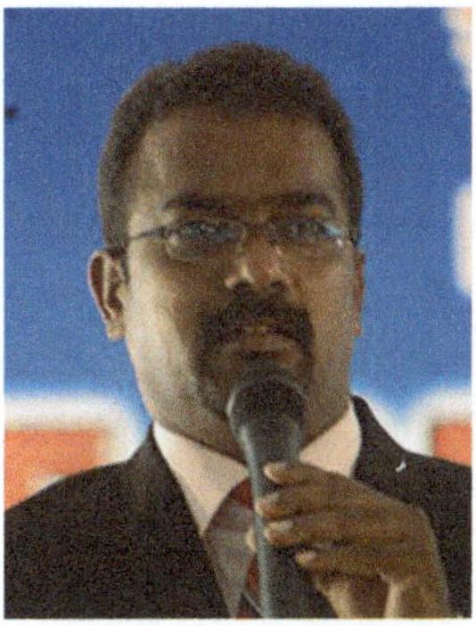

Emmanuel Janagan Johnson, MSW, MPhil, PhD, is a senior lecturer and chair in the Social Work Programme at the Department of Behavioural Sciences, the University of the West Indies, St. Augustine campus, in Trinidad. Dr. Johnson holds a PhD in Social Work, an M.Phil. in Social Work, an MA in Social Work, and a BA in English Literature from Bharathiar University, India. He has been teaching for over 26 years and has received several awards. Dr. Johnson's areas of specialization include social work education, qualitative research, social work with children and families, domestic violence, child abuse, and community health. He has published two books, and contributed to chapters in several books and articles in more than 60 international refereed journals. Dr. Johnson is currently involved in two research activities and has a research ID website: https://www.researchgate.net/profile/EmmanuelJohnson4.

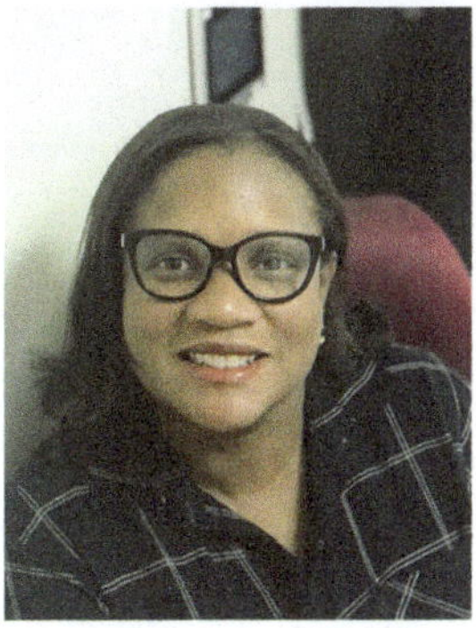

Camille L. Huggins, PhD, is a lecturer at the University of the West Indies, St. Augustine campus, in Trinidad. Her research interests include older adults, Caribbean culture, and social policy. Dr. Huggins obtained a master's in social work from Columbia University and a PhD in clinical social work from New York University, both located in New York, USA. She has been working with older adults in long-term care for eight years and has held various administrative positions. Dr. Huggins has presented papers at conferences and seminars, and contributed to several public, professional, and departmental service articles. She has published chapters in several books and articles in international refereed journals.

Chapter 1
The Unique Environment of the Caribbean

Important Highlights:

- Introduction to the various races and ethnicities currently living in the Caribbean.
- The importance of anti-oppressive practice in the Caribbean.

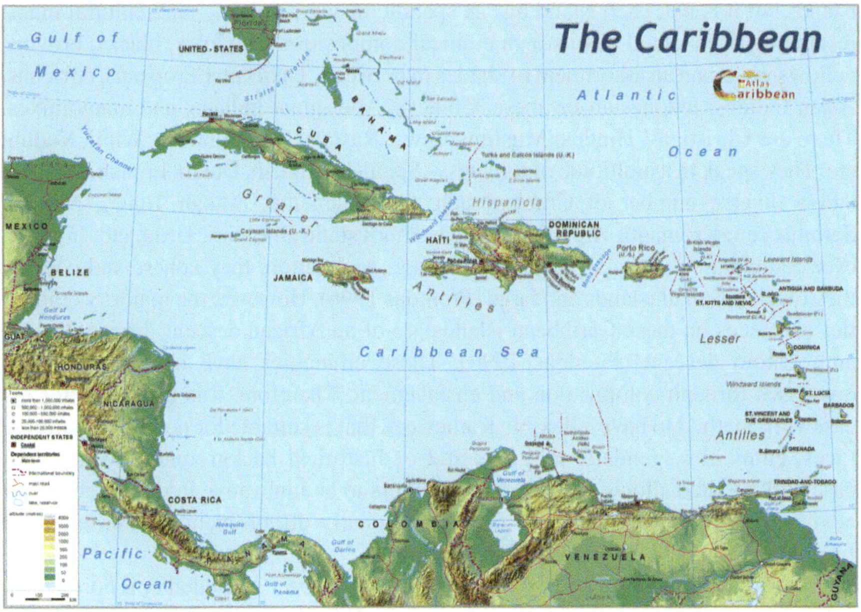

Courtesy: Google Maps

E. J. Johnson, C. L. Huggins, *Social Casework Methodology: A Skills Handbook for the Caribbean Human Services Worker*, SpringerBriefs in Social Work,
https://doi.org/10.1007/978-3-030-27319-4_1

Introduction to the Various Races and Ethnicities Currently Living in the Caribbean

The Caribbean sits in the cradle of the Americas (e.g. North, South and Central). It has always been a unique microcosm of the developed world with similar political, social and economic processes and systems. There are approximately 44 million people living on thirty islands (e.g., 13 sovereign states and 17 dependent states, Engerman 2000) speaking various languages such as, English, Spanish, French and Dutch to name a few. A sovereign state (or independent state) is responsible for their own people and governs themselves while dependent states do not exercise the full range of power over their own affairs and rely on a sovereign state to protect them economically. Since 1945 there has been strong international pressure to eliminate forms of dependency associated with colonialism (Brown 1963). The ethnicities, races, religions, and cultures of the Caribbean represent most of the developed nations of the world because every one of these nations has at one point in history transverse the Caribbean, leaving their imprint. Therefore, the Caribbean is very diverse with cultural practices and ethnicities.

In fact, the word the Caribbean may denote that it is one country unified by many islands but it is not, each island has its specific history, dialectic, and cultural manifestations. Each island has its own ethnical composition of whites, blacks, browns, yellows, reds, and an assortment of shades in between. There are Europeans, Africans, Asian Indians, Indonesian Javanese, Chinese, Aboriginal Indians, and many mixes. There are Christians, Hindus, Muslims, Jews, Rastafarians, Santería, Winti, Vudun, etc. They speak in a multitude of tongues—Spanish, English, Dutch, French, English, and a diverse number of Creoles such as Papiamentu, Sranan Tongo, Ndjuka, Saramaccan, Kromanti, Kreyol, as well as Hindustani, Bhojpuri, Urdu, etc. In whatever combinations of race, religion, language, and culture they cohere and coexist, they dwell on small islands and large (Premdas 1996). However, the majority ethnicities and races on these Caribbean islands are of an African descent, Indian descent and, Latino descent (Premdas 1996). These ethnicities have been traditionally oppressed through colonization and enslavement. Therefore, it is important for the casework method to have a flexible framework that is suitable for people of different races, ethnicities, genders, religions and or historical backgrounds. Social work casework method allows social service workers to be innovative in their methods of advocating for people who have been traditionally disenfranchised and excluded from accessing help (Bailey and Johnson 2014).

These disenfranchised and excluded persons have been excluded or ignored from receiving government assistance to the extent that they have developed their own coping mechanisms to survive whether it is beneficial (e.g., relying on the family) or negative (e.g., alcohol or drug abuse). These are people who have suffered from the shame and stigma from being discriminated against and as a result they are often insular within their own community on how they think, how they access resources and how they resolve issues even to their own detriment. So it is important to practice anti-oppressive social work.

The Importance of Anti-Oppressive Practice in the Caribbean

Anti-Oppressive Practice (AOP)

Anti-oppressive practice (AOP) is geared to raise social justice issues in order to improve the outcomes of the clients. The AOP lens is that of power based on group identities or affiliations (such as race, class, gender, and sexual identity), and when practitioners notice group identities, they can anticipate an array of experiences that are associated with positive or negative life outcomes (such as health, income, education, marginalization, violence, status, and social inclusion/exclusion). The simplest directive for AOP practice is to minimize power hierarchies, by assisting to build the power of those who hold a marginalized identity and/or reducing the unfair power of those of privileged status (Dominelli 2002).

The larger social and political context of the last generation that gave impetus to the emergence of AOP is the deepening of globalization and the rise of neoliberal policies, including cuts to social programs, rising inequality, and dominant discourse that blames individuals for their distress. In this deteriorating environment, social work has retained its divide of a more clinical orientation that is strongly aligned with counseling and psychology and a more social justice orientation to practice that focuses attention upstream on causal and contributing features to downstream distress. Anti-oppressive practice embodies a person-centered philosophy; an egalitarian value system concerned with reducing the deleterious effects of structural inequalities upon people's lives; a methodology focusing on both process and outcome; and a way of structuring relationships between individuals that aims to empower users by reducing the negative effects of hierarchy on their interaction and the work they do together (Dominelli 2002).

Although the Caribbean is similar to the developed world all of the islands hold the status as a 'developing' country where they have a less developed industrial economy (United Nations Statistical division 2018). Developing countries are characterized by having less access to proper amenities relating to health, shortage in water supply and, shortcomings in the area of medical supplies. These countries also experience higher birth rates and poor nutrition and as a result a higher susceptibility to natural diseases (e.g., infectious diseases) with eventual higher than normal death rates (Cox and Pawar 2013). Some countries are more developed than others because they have resources and a more developed industrial economy such as Trinidad (Butterfield and Cohen 2017). Many other Caribbean islands' government face the challenge of increasing their economic independence from larger developed countries.

Review Questions

1. What does the term anti-oppressive practice?
2. Name a few races and ethnicities that currently live in the Caribbean.

References

Bailey, K. R., & Johnson, E. J. (2014). Internet- based technologies in social work education: Experiences, perspectives and use. *The Caribbean Teaching Scholar Journal, 4*(1), 23–37.

Brown, M. B. (1963). *After imperialism*. London: Heinemann.

Butterfield, A., & Cohen, C. (2017). *Practicing as a social work educator in international collaboration*. Virginia: Council on Social Work Education, Inc.

Cox, D., & Pawar, M. (2013). *International social work: Issues, strategies and programs* (2nd ed.). Los Angeles: Sage Publications.

Dominelli, L. (2002). *Anti-oppressive social work theory and practice*. Basingstoke: Palgrave Macmillan.

Engerman, S. L. (2000). A population history of the Caribbean. In M. R. Haines & R. H. Steckel (Eds.), *A population history of North America* (pp. 483–528). Cambridge: Cambridge University Press.

Premdas, R. (Spring, 1996). *Ethnicity and development: The Caribbean and Oceania*. Working Paper #221. Kellogg Institute.

United Nations Statistical Commission. (2018, March). 49th session of the United Nations Statistical Commission on better data, better lives. https://unstats.un.org/unsd/statcom/.

Chapter 2
Social Problems in the Caribbean

Important Highlights:

- A review of prevalent social problems in the Caribbean.
- A highlight of the current social welfare systems in the Caribbean.
- An understanding of social welfare education in the Caribbean.

Social Problems

Review of Prevalent Social Problems in the Caribbean

Poverty

Caribbean countries have larger than normal pockets of poverty and related problems for decades. The Caribbean's small island economies face formidable challenges in dealing with globalization. Race, class and gender hierarchies of colonial domination have left a legacy of exclusion of the poor. Despite general improvements in living standards, poverty rates average 30% of the Caribbean population (UNEP 2008). Social and human development indicators show that Barbados, Antigua-Barbuda and the Bahamas are doing better than Belize, Dominica, Grenada, Jamaica, and Suriname. Plagued by political and economic problems, Haiti consistently scores lowest.

The causes and characteristics of poverty in the Caribbean are low educational attainment, the intergenerational transfer of poverty as well as, stigmatization and discrimination. Education plays a fundamental role in people's life trajectories and it is the principal mechanism for overcoming unequal social status that a person may be born into and level the playing field (Franco et al. 2011). In the Caribbean, educational attainment on a primary level may be achieved but there is

E. J. Johnson, C. L. Huggins, *Social Casework Methodology: A Skills Handbook for the Caribbean Human Services Worker*, SpringerBriefs in Social Work,
https://doi.org/10.1007/978-3-030-27319-4_2

still limited access to secondary and tertiary education for all people in the Caribbean whether it is access to a nearby learning institution or the intergenerational transfer of poverty.

Poverty is a complex set of positive and negative factors that affect an individual's chances of experiencing poverty, either in the present or at a future point in their life-course. The factors influencing an individual's likelihood of being poor include both the 'private' transmission (and lack of transmission) of capital and the 'public' transfer (or lack of transfer) of resources from one generation to the next (Bird 2010). Stigmatization and discrimination also contribute to poverty as a person or persons are excluded from participating in the general population due to an illness (e.g., HIV/AIDS). There are also the historical structural effects of racism, cultural and ethnic battles for dominance are often played out here in Caribbean politics. Islands such as the Dominican Republic, the poorest half of the population receives less than one-fifth of the Gross National Product while the richest 10% benefit from 40% of the national income (The World Bank 2014).

There is also factors that contribute to extreme poverty (e.g., Haiti) such as political corruption, the 'brain drain' (e.g., educated citizens leaving the country for more developed countries), business monopolies, deforestation, decreased tourism and the economic embargo for specific countries (e.g., Cuba, UNEP 2008).

Human Trafficking

The act of trafficking a person includes the recruitment, transportation, transfer, or harbouring someone by means of threat or force or other forms of coercion, or abduction, or by fraudulent means, or deception, or the abuse of power or of a position of vulnerability or of the giving or receiving of payments or benefits to achieve the consent of a person having control over another person, for the purpose of exploitation. Exploitation shall include, at a minimum, the exploitation of the prostitution of others or other forms of sexual exploitation, forced labor or services, slavery or practices similar to slavery, servitude or the removal of organs (United Nations Office on Drug and Crime 2018).

In the Caribbean human trafficking may begin or be a point of origin where the person may be abducted and then shipped to another county such as to the United States or to Venezuela, a transhipment point where the person is brought from another country (e.g., Columbia) to the Caribbean temporarily and then sent to the intended country (e.g., Canada) or as a final destination point where the person is transferred from another country and brought to the Caribbean to stay permanently (Amesty International 2016). With regards to drug trafficking, the Caribbean is also a point of origin (e.g., Marijuana) as well as a trans-shipment point (e.g., cocaine) from South to North America. Sixteen percent of all cocaine that is transported to the United States comes through the Caribbean.

Crime and Drugs

With high levels of unemployment and the persistent presence of poverty in the Caribbean islands, it is a huge trans-shipment route for drugs heading to the United States which has resulted in high rates of violence and gang-related crime. Youths aged 25 years or younger living in the Caribbean are usually responsible for 52% of arrests for total major crimes in 2005 (52% of murders; 59% of shootings; 54% of robberies).

In the 1980s, the Caribbean Sea was the preferred route for Latin America's drug traffickers, with around 80% of all US-bound cocaine transiting through the region. It slowed down for a period due to anti-narcotic operations in the Caribbean but in 2013, cocaine flow to the United States via the Caribbean reportedly reached its highest levels in a decade. There are large amounts of cocaine and marijuana in transit through the Dominican Republic, Haiti, Jamaica, Trinidad and Tobago, The Bahamas, the Dutch Caribbean (e.g., Antiqua) and the Eastern Caribbean (e.g., St. Kitts) to the United States.

The illegal drug trade has fuelled high levels of violence in the Caribbean region. In Puerto Rico, for example, at least 80% of killings are believed to be drug-related. The region continues to see local gang wars over control of criminal economies and is characterized by high gun use. There are an estimated 1.6 million illegal firearms circulating in the Caribbean.

Access to Health Care and Ageing

Health care systems in the Caribbean need improvement and strengthening by the way of health care systems and personnel. Although some Caribbean islands pronounce health care is free and accessible to the public, what is available is extended waiting times to see a physician or specialist, lack of medication and limited services for cancer care or other related diseases. In the Caribbean most people or eight of 10 deaths are due to non-communicable diseases (NCDs, e.g., diabetes, heart disease, strokes). Diabetes, ischaemic heart disease and strokes are among the top three causes of death in the Caribbean. The estimated lifetime cancer risk is 18%; 20% for men and 16% for women. Prostate, breast, colorectal and cervical cancer are the commonest types of preventable cancer. Cervical cancer is the most preventable, yet in many countries, only half the women have had a cervical cancer screening test. There are also threats of contagious diseases all over the world, like Chikungunya and Ebola. These threats also pose potentially negative effects on the tourism sector in the Caribbean. High and middle-income population may get their health care from abroad or the private sector while the poorest rely on the public system. Most citizens have to pay out of pocket expenditures to get the most rudimentary health care assistance (Caribbean Public Health Agency 2015). Threats to health posed by extreme weather events in the Caribbean include insect- and rodent-borne diseases,

Table 2.1 Life expectancy in the Caribbean

Attributes	Guyana	Jamaica	Trinidad & Tobago	All Caribbean
Population age 60+	6.9	11.5% (Older Persons in Jamaica 2012)	13% (Central statistical office 2011)	9.9
Life expectancy				
Women	66.0	77.0	77.2	70.9
Men	58.0	73.0	72.5	65.4
% in poverty	35	19	21	28

such as dengue, leptospirosis, malaria and yellow fever; water-borne diseases, including schistosomiasis, cryptosporidium and cholera; food-borne diseases, including diarrhea, food poisoning, salmonellosis and typhoid; respiratory diseases, including asthma, bronchitis and respiratory allergies and infections; and malnutrition resulting from food production or distribution disruptions.

Although Caribbean people are living longer the life expectancy is still 6–8 years shorter than in developed countries (e.g., Japan, Switzerland) (Table 2.1).

Older adults in the Caribbean have trouble with their quality of life due to retirement some may not receive little to no compensation from the government or from a pension. About one-third of those older than 60 years are greater than 75 years. One in three men and one in six women over 60 years old are in the workforce but experience regular income-insecurity (Palloni and McEniry 2007). Disability in this age group is four times higher than the general population, particularly for women. There is also a higher burden of all chronic diseases (e.g., diabetes, hypertension, Alzheimer's) among the elderly. It is also a high risk for older people becoming poor because of disability. A high portion of Caribbean people work in the informal sector (i.e., domestic, entrepreneurship) and did not pay into the pension program.

Some older adults may have issues with intergenerational relations where the younger generation (e.g., children, grandchildren) may not be able to care for them as they did traditionally because the younger generation is working more or emigrate and older adults are left with irregular family support. Many older adults live in urban areas in the Caribbean but about 30% still live in rural communities with little access to services and appropriate living conditions. Overall, access to quality health care and aging are problematic in the Caribbean and there is little information about the circumstances of older adults which may hinder policy development and services.

These are just a few of the social problems that plague the Caribbean there are a myriad of others such as; child abuse, domestic violence and issues that have grown in the advent of globalization such as; instability in economic and government structures (e.g., corruption, oil, tourism), and the remnants of colonization. It is important to keep in mind these social problems are specific to the environment and should be assessed and evaluated for the unique Caribbean environment so the intervention can be mutually understood and agreed upon by the social service worker and the client(s).

Natural Disasters: Climate Change

Caribbean countries generally consist of island states, the exceptions being Belize in Central America, and Guyana and Suriname, situated on the South American continent. The topography is generally rugged and mountainous with small areas of flat land in coastal areas. Several islands are volcanic in origin, while others are comprised primarily of coral. Many Caribbean islands rely almost entirely on a single source of water such as groundwater, imports, rainwater, surface reservoirs, rivers and other surface flows. In islands such as Anguilla, Antigua and Barbuda, Grenada, and Barbados, more than 65% of total annual rainfall may be recorded in the wet season from June to December (UNEP 2008).

The Caribbean region is vulnerable to natural hazards (e.g. hurricanes, earthquakes, tsunamis and volcanic eruptions); deforestation, which over time reduce intrinsic ecosystem resilience; transport of toxic waste; and global climate change, the effects of which are particularly severe on small island states (UNEP 2008). Serious vulnerability to extreme climate events (e.g., shifting rainfall patterns and cyclones, typhoons and hurricanes) and other natural disasters. Environmental vulnerability is related to the risk of damage to a country's natural capital. Caribbean islands are susceptible to the effects of climate change with rising sea levels and extreme meteorological events (e.g., extreme rainstorms), economic and social vulnerability.

In the Caribbean, production is heavily dependent on their limited natural resource base (e.g., agriculture, forestry, fishing, tourism) and scarce land resources. The major foreign exchange earning sectors and employers are mining, tourism, agriculture and offshore banking, all of which are very likely to be disrupted by extreme meteorological events of which hurricanes are the most common. There is also increased pressure on coastal and marine environments and resources to trade and export as a result there is limited ability to develop economies of scale. There is also a limited ability for economic diversification possibilities. Tourism is also a major and most rapidly growing industry across the region. Mining and mineral extraction industries, located principally in the larger islands, are also important engines of economic growth and development. As well as, mining is an important sector in some Caribbean countries. Guyana, Jamaica, and Trinidad and Tobago accounting for respectively, 19.3%, 7.9% and 10.6% of gross domestic product (GDP) in the

Caribbean region. In Jamaica, the bauxite-alumina industry is one of the most important economic earners. Gold, diamond, and bauxite mining are important in Guyana (gold, diamond, bauxite). The Dominican Republic is also an exporter of ferronickel and gold.

Natural disasters and unfavorable weather have also caused major damage to infrastructure and have further increased economic pressures (Johnson 2014). For example, in August 2017 Hurricane Irma, Puerto Rico, Barbuda, and St. Maarten were devastated. Virtually all the major tourism facilities located along the coast were ruined and resulted in closures and lost revenue. These phenomena have put a huge amount of the region's resources at risk, including coastal infrastructure, human settlements, utilities and coastal ecosystems (e.g. mangroves, seagrass beds, and coral reefs).

Social Welfare Systems in the Caribbean

Social Welfare programs were essentially brought to the Caribbean via colonialism and Christian centered organizations. Its main purpose was to meet the needs and objectives of those in power. Those who colonialized for all extensive purposes truly believed they were bringing a kind of civility to their captured territories and social welfare services were established to reflect this objective. Social welfare and social workers were historically recruited from the colonial home country to govern the organization and any support staff was formally trained in the colonized way of operations. In a number of colonies, training regarding social welfare and community development were introduced as more and more local people were recruited to staff the developing social service agencies and systems. Local-born social service workers although few were chosen via a scholarship to study abroad in the colonizer's country. Once the local-born social service worker returned they were assigned to work in rural and disparate locations where the foreign-born workers were hesitant to venture.

The purpose of the social welfare systems was to emphasize health, education and law and order in accordance with the colonizers. The social welfare organizations usually catered to classes whose roles were deemed important to the colonial system, with the needs of many others ignored (Cox and Pawar 2013). Those that were not in the sphere of these programs would receive services that were not necessary to meet their welfare and developmental needs but to civilize and Christianize individuals. The mindset was if the population were civilized and Christian they would be able to meet their own needs (Hoogvelt 2001).

Post-colonization, in the 1950s and 1960s the United Nations established a stance for the development of professional social work and social welfare in developing nations. As per the United Nations Social Welfare Commission (UNSWC) an organization promoting social development across the world. It is the mandate to provide substantive support to Governments in developing policy measures and initiatives to promote inclusive "societies for all", where each individual has rights and responsibilities regardless of economic status (poverty), social status (gender, marital), specific age group (older persons, youth), disability or cultural or religious affiliation. The aim is to ensure that individuals and communities are enabled to participate in society and contribute to national development while enjoying basic human rights and fundamental freedoms (United National Department of Economic and Social Affairs 2011). The United Nations felt those countries that were not colonized were affected by colonialism because some were not allowed to participate in economic trade between countries (i.e., Haiti) and did not benefit in developing their country and the quality of life of its people (Cox and Pawar 2013). Another perspective of the United Nations was although colonialism involved imposing Western standards in the developing world it at least laid a foundation for modern social welfare and social work developments. The reality that a number of developing countries who did not establish and maintain a state-run social services or modern social work practice were categorized as least developing countries with limited hope of survival of its people long term (Cox and Pawar 2013).

Social welfare programs provide basic services but there is little provision for the able-bodied. Maintaining the poor at the threshold of poverty may be valued politically in some areas. Social safety net programs such as national insurance, food stamps, and student loans aim to target resources where they are needed most. Though forming the mainstay of publicly funded programs in the Caribbean, they serve to alleviate rather than reduce poverty.

Social Welfare Education in the Caribbean

Social work and human services education established during the post-colonial period in the Caribbean often framed its philosophical underpinning and curriculum from American and British models of professional social work. There are some positives to this approach as the American and British models are the architects of the social welfare and social work philosophy. These models provide the technical assistance and principles and those countries that have emulated these systems to some degree have advanced in the welfare of its people and the production of its industries and economy (Cox and Pawar 2013). However social problems and helping people change behavior is embedded in the culture and social-political practices. No longer are colonizers available to enforce proper health, education and law and order practices. The advent of *free will* infused with societal practices, there is no mechanism to make individuals comply with behavior modification even if it is for their own good. The belief that Eurocentric, knowledge-based profession of social welfare and social work can apply to any part of the world, regardless of the diverse social practices, beliefs and culture has been proven to be false because of its failings as a profession in parts of India and Africa (George and Krishankumar 2014; Olaleye 2013). For example, in India, professional social work emerged as a profession in 1936 but has failed to gain social recognition because it has not responded effectively to local social issues such as; poverty, suicide, child labor (George and Krishankumar 2014).

Indigenous social work education and practice draw its inspiration and nourishment from society but it, in turn, contributes to the growth renewal and development of that society. In developing countries, the cultural paradigms through which indigenous knowledge is transmitted differ significantly from American and British cultural models of education and ways of knowing of being and doing. Indigenous methods of social work practice, pedagogy and epistemologies are an important aspect of social work practice in the Caribbean. Cultural or indigenous knowledge of society is fundamentally based upon the transgenerational transmission of culture and knowledge (Olaleye 2013). Indigenous Caribbean education and knowledge have generally been understood as a simplistic process of socialization involving the preparation of children for work in the home, the village and within an ethnic domain. To be a professional social service worker in the Caribbean 'knowledge about how the indigenous context affects the relationship between individuals and their surrounding is essential. The social work method framework provides the room for indigenous practice within the worker-client-environment model paradigm.

The textbooks for schools in non-Western countries are also not reflective of developing countries social welfare systems and especially not indicative of the Caribbean. American and British models of professional social work are unable to address the unique needs and cultural characteristics of the Caribbean. These textbooks do not include the cultural patterns of problem-solving for local communities and how knowledge is shared and dispersed into the communities' understanding (Olaleye 2013). Most textbooks are from the West; course instruction and theories discussed in the classroom focused on their applicability to Western countries rather than to Caribbean's social context. This has developed a chasm between the local social issues and needs and what the local social welfare and social worker is trained to deal with. Local social issues in the Caribbean like poverty, suicide, mental health issues and violence against children and women are not clearly understood and dealt with because of cultural differences of what is taught in the classroom and what is seen in the community (George and Krishnakumar 2014).

A Way Forward

It is estimated that over 44 million people live in the Caribbean which includes island countries within the Caribbean Sea, from Cuba to the north and Trinidad and Tobago to the south which includes the Bahamas, though it is not geographically within the Caribbean, along with Belize, Suriname and Guyana (United Nations Department of Economic and Social Affairs 2017). Most of the Caribbean islands have high levels of poverty and all the ailments that attribute to poverty. There is some form in varying degrees of the social welfare system in every Caribbean island with fragile institutional structures (Cloos et al. 2009). Most Caribbean islands have burgeoning social welfare systems that are developed at the discretion of government or if there is an immediate social ill that must be addressed. Many small islands have child welfare organizations and social welfare systems that do not address the majority of the needs of the population.

The social welfare and social work interventions and theories must be effective to work with the people. It should also be a support of the welfare state. The government should participate in dictating the specific interventions for any field of practice, as most social service workers are employed directly by the government. This will promote elements of social control by the government and protection of vulnerable populations.

Professional social welfare education in the Caribbean should be committed to enhancing the social functioning or well-being of individuals and families by working directly with clients experiencing problems (Cox and Pawar 2013; Johnson et.al 2012). Workers should always be committed to working with and on the behalf of the individuals in the areas where they are most in need such as; hospitals, youth detention centers, and prisons. Social Welfare and social workers should also seek to contribute to the building of healthy, cohesive and enabling communities and societies and by the process of promoting the well-being of people. The fields of practice in this area range from community development to macro social policy formulation. The goal of community work is to improve the environment or societies where people develop and live (George and Krishnakumar 2014).

This approach is in line with creating a pro-community and individual approach to social welfare and social work that is stipulated in the International Federation of Social Work Ethics (IFSW 2014) concerning an approach that might facilitate constructive confrontation and change where certain cultural beliefs, values, and traditions violate peoples' basic human rights and community building.

Social casework method is one such method that is the art of doing different things for and with different people by cooperating with them to achieve at one and the same time their own and society's betterment (Mary Richmond 1917). Social Casework is concerned with the adjustment and development of the individual towards a more satisfying human relationship. It is a method to provide a better family life, improved schools, better housing, more hospitals, and medical care facilities, protected economic conditions and better relations between racial, religious and cultural groups. Social casework method fits the environment because it is concerned about the individual as well as society as a whole. Social Casework, a primary method of social work, is not only concerned with the adjustment and development of the individual towards more satisfying human relations.

Review Questions

1. Name an important social problem that is relevant to the Caribbean.
2. What kind of skills do you need to work in the Caribbean as a social service worker?
3. Why is it so important to understand the social problems in the Caribbean as opposed to other social environments?

References

Amnesty International. (2016). Amnesty International Annual Report 2015/2016. WWW.AMNESTY.ORG/EN/LATEST/RESEARCH/2016/02/ANNUAL-REPORT-201516/.

Bird, K. (2010). The intergenerational transmission of poverty: An overview. *Chronic poverty research centre working paper, No. 99*. p. 63.

Caribbean Public Health Agency. (2015). Preventing disease, promoting and protecting health.

Central Statistical Office (2011). *2911 Housing and Population Census*. Trinidad and Tobago: Trinidad and Tobago Ministry of Planning and Sustainable Development.

Cloos, P., Allen, C., Alvarado, B., & Zunzunegui, M. (2009). Active ageing: A qualitative study in six Caribbean countries. *Aging and Society, 30*(1), 79–101. https://doi.org/10.1017/S0144686X09990286.

Cox, D., & Pawar, M. (2013). *International social work: Issues, strategies and programs* (2nd ed.). Los Angeles: Sage Publications.

Eldemire-shearer, D.; James, K., Waldron, N.; Mitchell-Fearon, K. (2012). Older Persons in Jamaica 2012. Mona: University of the West Indies-Mona Campus.

Franco, R., Hopenhayn, M., & Leon, A. (2011). The growing and changing middle class in Latin America: An update. *Cepal Review, 103*, 7–25.

George, M., & Krishnakumar, I. (2014). Revisiting the landscape of professional social work in India. *Social Development Issues, 2*, 53–64.

Hoogvelt, A. (2001). *Globalization and the postcolonial world: The new political economy of development*. Maryland: John Hopkins University Press.

International Federation of Social Work. (2014). Global definition of social work. http://ifsw.org/policies/definition-of-social-work/.

Johnson, E. J. (2014). A case study on the impact of natural Disaster on 'Women'. *Asian Journal of Environment and Disaster Management, 6*(1, 1), –11.

Johnson, E. J., Bailey, K. R., & Padmore, J. (2012). Issues and challenges of social work practicum in Trinidad and Tobago and India. *The Caribbean Teaching Scholar, 2*(1), 19–29.

Olaleye, Y. (2013). Indigenous cultural practices as precursors to social work education in Nigeria. *IFE PsychologIA: An International Journal, 21*, 2106–2112.

Palloni, A., & Mc Eniry, M. (2007). Aging and health status of elderly in Latin America and the Caribbean: Preliminary findings. *Journal of Cross-Cultural Gerontology, 22*(3), 263–285.

Richmond, M. (1917). *Social diagnosis*. New York: Russell Sage Foundation.

United National Department of Economic and Social Affairs. (2011). *Sustainable development goals*. www.un.org/development/desa/en/

United Nations Department of Economic and Social Affairs. (2017). World population prospects: The 2017 revision. ESA.UN.org.

United Nations Environment Programme Regional Office for Latin America and the Caribbean. (2008). *Climate change in the Caribbean and the challenge of adaptation*. Panama City: United Nations Environment Programme.

United Nations Office on Drug and Crime. (2018). *What is Human Trafficking?* https://www.unodc.org/unodc/en/human-trafficking/what-is-human-trafficking.html.

World Bank. (2014). *The World Bank Annual Report 2014*. Washington, DC. World Bank. https://openknowledge.worldbank.org/handle/10986/20093 License: CC BY-NC-ND 3.0 IGO.

Chapter 3
History of the Social Casework Method

Important Highlights:

- A review of the history of the casework method.
- An introduction to the important contributors in creating the casework method.
- A definition of the casework method.
- An overview of the principles of the casework method.

The Beginning of Casework Methods

Though casework is a mode of helping people on the basis of a person-to-person relationship was present in every society from ancient times, the professional method of casework originated in the U.S.A. in the second decade of this century. One of the earliest organized efforts in the U.S.A. to help the poor was the establishment of the American Charity Organization Society in 1877 on the pattern of the Charity Organization of London, which was started 7 years earlier. One of the aims of the society was to find out ways and means of helping the poor and needy and thus to organise individualized services geared to this purpose. The society used volunteers, who were called friendly visitors, to visit the homes of the poor for purposes of assessing their need, for rendering material assistance and for giving them guidance and advice. The friendly visitors were subsequently supplemented by 'paid agents'. These paid helpers gradually developed, systematic procedures in performing their tasks. They collected data about needy individuals and families and helped them after assessing their need. They also maintained records in which they kept all the information including personal data, as well as the type of help rendered. It was out of the practice of these early workers that casework developed gradually to a professional method in subsequent years. Their collective experience of knowing the poor families and their problems and the concurrent studies of poverty by social scientists broadened the understanding of human behavior. There was

E. J. Johnson, C. L. Huggins, *Social Casework Methodology: A Skills Handbook for the Caribbean Human Services Worker*, SpringerBriefs in Social Work,
https://doi.org/10.1007/978-3-030-27319-4_3

the growing recognition that there were forces within the individual and forces external to him which influenced his behavior and the nature of his existence in society. In course of time, the terms 'paid agents'and 'the poor' were supplanted by caseworkers and clients respectively in the terminology of the help giving organization and the office of the organization came to be known as the agency.

There are always been some form of casework method when working with the disadvantaged in every society because of the simplicity of the approach and the positive outcomes. The professionalized method of casework originated in the U.S.A. in the early part of the twentieth century. One of the earliest social welfare organizations opened in the U.S.A. was the American Charity Organization Society (ACOS) in 1877. The ACOS was patterned after the Charity Organization of London, which started 7 years earlier (Bosanquet 1914). The aims of the ACOS was to find out ways and means of helping the poor and needy with organized individualized services.

The ACOS used volunteers, who were called "friendly visitors", to visit the homes of the poor for purposes of assessing their needs (e.g., parenting advise, housekeeping practices), rendering material assistance and giving them guidance and advice (Richmond 1917). The "friendly visitors" were subsequently supplemented by 'paid agents'. These paid helpers gradually developed, systematic procedures in performing their tasks. Data was collected and maintained about individuals and families that were helped, the progress the individuals and families made after receiving the help and what services were needed subsequently. It was out of the practice of these early workers that casework developed gradually into a professional method (Bosanquet 1914). In time the terms 'paid agents'and 'the poor' were supplanted with new terms of 'caseworkers' and 'clients' respectively and the 'charitable organization' came to be known as the 'agency.' The workers of the ACOS studied the collective experience of poor families with their problems while nationwide concurrent studies on poverty conducted by social scientists in the U.S. an understanding of human behavior was created. There was a growing recognition that there were forces within the individual and forces outside of the individual which influenced behavior.

The initial theories helped to develop the science of fact gathering, the methodology for making judgments about whether and how to give help. The years to follow, some casework theoreticians began to examine sociological concepts like social role, social system, social class, with reference to their applicability to casework situations. The result was the shifting of the focus from the self of the individual to the self and the person's social settings.

Mary Richmond's book, **Social Diagnosis,** published in 1917, is considered the first book in casework. It provided a methodology of helping clients through systematic ways of assessing their problems and handling each problem systematically. The book introduced the principle of individualization and also acknowledged the client's right to self-determination. While Richmond (1917) viewed environmental conditions as crucial in affecting individuals, she also viewed each person as unique in the way he or she dealt with these social factors. According to Richmond (1917), the techniques of the casework method suggested more rational approaches to dealing with clients.

The first training program for caseworkers was in the form of summer courses but as the need grew there was a need for more substantial training and schools of social work, attached to agencies. When these schools attained a certain standing in the community, they were recognized as professional schools under the administrative authority of universities.

Casework Method Definition

The social casework method is one of the primary approaches to social welfare practice. Early iterations of the definition defined it as an adjustment and development of the individual towards a more satisfying human relationship with others (Richmond 1917). It is an individualistic approach for helping the person improve: their family life, peer relationships, housing conditions, access to health care through hospitals, and the person's overall economic conditions. This method evaluates the person's resources whether it's internal (e.g., self-determination and abilities) or the external resources (e.g., access to services and supports). It is concerned with methods to assist the social service worker to first study the problem, then make an assessment or diagnosis of it and create a solution and help the client work towards it.

The nature of the casework relationship is the development of security and acceptance fostered by the casework practitioner with the client in the casework relationship which enables clients to engage in the often painful process of the helping relationship. Even in settings where the focus is not on changes in self and/or relationships, such as medical services, many heavy emotional issues are involved, including clients' feelings related to loss, rejection, diminishing the sense of body integrity and fear of death. Social service workers must learn how to be caring, accepting and empathic in professional ways, without immersing themselves in the life of the client, becoming frightened by the client's emotions, or feeling totally responsible for 'fixing' the client's problems. The casework method is a potential minefield of problems the client will share and the complex relationship the social service worker will face with regards to the client (Urdang 2010).

Utilizing the social casework method helps the worker work collaboratively with the individual to understand the client's circumstances and make adjustments to meet their goals. This is accomplished in a dyadic (i.e., one to one) relationship with a careful examination of social functioning, interpersonal relationships, and social roles. It is concerned with an informed understanding of the present more complex social conditions and the role that individuals are expected to play in it and the help they may need to do so (Urdang 2010).

Other social work pioneers contributed to the definition of the casework method and utilized this method to develop other social welfare fields such as child welfare, gerontology, medical and psychiatric social work (National Association of Social Worker Foundation 2004).

The psychosocial casework models of Hamilton and Hollis in the 1950s and 1960s attempted, through the incorporation of the person-in-environment concept (Hollis and Woods 1981), to promote an approach to social work that (1) focused on both individual and environmental problems and (2) focused on both weaknesses or deficits and strengths.

Mary Richmond (1861–1928) was an American social work pioneer stated in (1915) "Social Casework may be defined as the Art of doing different things with different people, co-operating with them to achieve some of their own & society's betterment."

Mary Richmond stated in (1917) "Social casework is the art of bringing about better adjustments in the social relationship of individual men or women or children."

Mary Richmond stated in (1922) "Social casework means, processes which develop personality through adjustment or consciously affecting, individual by individual, and their social environment."

Mary Cromwell Jarrett (1877–1961) the founder of psychiatric social work stated in (1919) social casework is "the art of bringing an individual who is in a condition of social disorder into the best possible relationship with all parts of his environment".

Jessie Taft (1882–1960) developed the first American authority on child placement and therapeutic interventions for children stated in (1920). Social casework means "social treatment of a maladjusted individual involving an attempt to understand his personality, behavior and social relationships and to assist him in working out better social and personal adjustment".

John Broadus Watson, (1879–1958), an American psychologist who is considered the father of the psychological school of behaviorism stated in (1922) "Social casework is the art of untangling and restructuring the twisted personality in such a manner that the individual can adjust himself to his environment."

Ethel Lee a young social worker for the Charity Organization Society who bought hope to those living in poverty and suffering from tuberculosis stated in (1923) "Social casework is the art of changing human attitudes"

Ruth Taylor, a social work pioneer and medical social work consultant who joined the Public Health Service Tuberculosis Control Program in its early years stated in (1926) "Social casework is a process concerned with the understanding of individuals as whole personalities and with the adjustments of these socially healthy lives."

Bertha Reynolds (1885–1978) social work pioneer stated in (1935) "Social casework is the process of counseling with a client on a problem which is essentially his own, involving some difficulty in his social relationships."

Bertha Reynolds in (1935) **"**Social casework is that form of social work which assists the individual to relate himself to his family, his natural group and, his community."

Elizabeth DeSchweiinitz (1895–1978) devoted to social welfare and provided instruction on social casework stated in (1939) "Casework means those processes involved in giving service, financial assistance, or personal counsel to individuals by the representatives of social agencies, according to polices established and with consideration of individual need."

Joseline and Pauline Strode (1948) wrote the first Introduction to social work textbook stated**:** "casework is the process of assisting the individual to the best possible social adjustment through the use of social case study, social resources and knowledge from relative fields of learning."

Charlotte Towle (1896–1966) created the geriatric casework curriculum stated in (1947) "Social casework is one method….by which certain social services are made available in areas of unmet needs."

Frank Swithun Bowers (1908–1992) a Canadian, wrote the nature and definition of social casework in 1949 stated "Social casework is an art in which knowledge of the sciences of human relations and skill in relationship are used to mobilize capacities in the individual and resources in the community appropriate for better adjustment between the client and all or any part of his total environment."

Florence Hollis (1907–1980) conducted pioneering work in her writing in social work education. Her last book, Casework: A Psychosocial Therapy stated in (1954) "Social casework is a method employed by the social worker to help individuals find a solution to problems of social adjustment which they are unable to handle in a satisfactory way by their own efforts."

(Amy) Gordon Hamilton (1892–1967) social work educator for School of Social Work at Columbia University stated in (1956) "Social casework (which is both a tool and area of work) consists of those processes which develop personality through adjustment consciously affected, individual by individual between man and his social environment." In social casework the client is stimulated to participate in the study of his situation, to share plans, to make an effective effort to solve his problems, using his own resources and whatever community resources are available and appropriate.

Helen Harris Perlman (1906–2004) joined the faculty of the School of Social Service Administration, University of Chicago, in 1945 and later became the Distinguished Service Professor Emerita stated in (1957) "Social casework is a process used by certain human welfare agencies to help individuals to cope more effectively with their problems in social functioning."

Virginia Satir (1916–1988) in 1976 she received a special alumni medal from the University of Chicago for her outstanding work in family therapy and human relationships stated "Social casework is a method employed by a social worker to help individual, find a solution to their problem of social adjustment which they are unable to handle in a satisfactory way by their own effort."

Rev. Felix Biestek (1912–1994) was an American priest and professor who made significant contributions to the field of social work during its period of expansion following World War- II. Biestek wrote extensively about the casework relationship and outlined seven principles regarding the casework relationship.

Individualization The recognition of each client as a unique individual. It is based on the need and the right of each human being to be treated as an individual and not just as a typical member of a category or group.

Purposeful Expression of Feeling The recognition of the client's need to express his feelings freely, especially his negative feelings. The worker listens purposefully, neither discouraging nor condemning the expression of these feelings. To deny a client the opportunity to express his feelings, his fears, his hopes, his hostility, etc. is a refusal to deal with the total person. In social work, it is believed that every problem or request for help has an emotional component and that the client has a need and right to express it.

Controlled Emotional Involvement The worker's sensitivity to the client's feelings, an understanding of the meaning of these feelings, and purposeful, appropriate response. The worker's response is not only verbal; it is also nonverbal. The worker becomes "involved" emotionally by sensing and responding to feelings. The involvement is "controlled" by the self-discipline of the worker, the purpose of the case, and other factors. This principle is one of the key principles in social work

Acceptance The worker perceives and deals with the client as he really is, including his strengths and weaknesses, his positive and negative feelings, his constructive and destructive attitudes and behavior, while maintaining and communicating a sense of the client's innate dignity and personal worth. Acceptance does not mean approval. The object of acceptance is not "the good", but "the real". The acceptance, which the client perceives, permits him to reveal himself fully, without damage to his sense of dignity.

Non-Judgmental Attitude The non-judgmental attitude is based on the belief that social work does not include assigning guilt or innocence. If the client fears blame and judgment, he will not talk about himself. Not only blame but also praise and approval, are examples of a judgmental attitude. Blame and praise may have the same effect on a client: to hide a part of himself so as not to be judged.

Client Self-Determination The recognition of the right and the need of the client to have freedom in making his own choices and decisions in the social work process. The worker does not take responsibility for the client, does not persuade in a controlling way, and does not manipulate the client to make decisions to conform to the worker's preferences. (The client's right to self-determination may be limited by the client's capacity for decision-making, by the civil and moral law, and by the function of the agency).

Confidentiality Confidentiality is the preservation of private information concerning the client, which is disclosed within the professional relationship, or is received from other sources in the course of working with a client. (The client's right to confidentiality is not absolute. There are situations in which another right or duty is greater than the client's right to confidentiality).

All these definitions explain some aspect of the casework method. Some definitions discuss casework is an art, which means it is a nuanced and creative approach to dealing with people, understanding their needs and solving their problems.

The worker must be perceptive, intuitive and able to handle multiple situations simultaneously. Other definitions touch on the environment including socio-economic and cultural factors impact on a client's behavior which means all humans are conditioned and influenced by their environment. Additional definitions of the casework method convey humans cannot grow and develop if certain basic needs are not met such as the physical, emotional, and intellectual development of the person. The basic physical needs refer to food, shelter and clothing and the emotional and intellectual needs are love, support, and trust. In all the casework method definition covers many aspects of human relationships and the techniques to help those in need.

Principles of the Social Casework Method

The principles of casework method guide the performance of the caseworker. Principles are rules that take into account the particular context of an act.

The first principle is **individualization.** Each case should be viewed with an open mind and a freshness of approach. In the casework method, each person is perceived as unique. It is important to be perceptively observant and visibly ready to respond to clients' particular needs in order to see the client as a distinct individual.

The second principle in the casework method is **acceptance** and a non-condemning or a non-judgmental attitude. Acceptance of the client regardless of their good and bad qualities, strengths and weaknesses, or behavior. Although the worker is a representative of society and should uphold the laws of the land there is an emphasis on the idea in which the offender needs help, before, during and after the process of a verdict. The worker understands the person who perpetrates the crime is acceptable as a person, though the crime is not. It is important to have the appropriate attitude of a professional that is friendly, benevolent and a willingness and desire to be of help.

The third principle is the **self-determination** of the casework method. Self-determination refers to the self-direction of an individual who has the right to make decisions about matters pertaining to their life and that other people's decisions about directing their life should not be imposed. In the dyadic (one on one) relationship in the casework method the worker should not make decisions alone but in collaboration with the client. The client makes their own decisions and the client must be willing to participate in the handling of the problem. The decision made by the clients should not be harmful to oneself and others and every decision the client makes is their responsibility to carry out the decision and handle the consequences. The process of helping and being helped does not stop at the point of decision making by the client, but it goes much further in terms of plans pursued and actions taken.

The last principle of casework method is **confidentiality.** Every worker is expected to maintain confidentiality regarding the information received from the client. It is important that the information which the client gives is taken and treated seriously. It is difficult to maintain confidentiality in the Caribbean because most communities are small, rural, with tightly interrelated systems of formal and informal social and political entities (Hargrove 1986). Relationships among community members are interdependent; complex; and may have deep historical, social, political, and familial roots (Helbok 2010). Members of the community often have multiple roles within the community, tend to rely on each other and on kinship ties, and prefer to take care of their own problems so confidentiality is often a foreign term that is not readily understood and carried out in a professional fashion.

Explanations of the Principles of Social Casework

- A worker should believe in social reality.
- Every individual has his own different problems because every personality is unique
- Problems do exist and there is no stigma attached to a problem and or any maladjusted person and a social worker do not believe in social isolation for the physically, mentally, emotionally and socially sick person.
- Every problem can, therefore, be solved provided we create conditions for an individual who helps to make an adjustment with his social environment.
- The personality of the client is to be respected.
- The worker should build up a purposeful relationship with the client.
- The worker should always have a belief in the ability of human beings to change and grow.
- The worker should not involve himself emotionally with the client. There should not be any over-identification with the client
- The worker has to accept and appreciate the individual differences and prejudices of the client.
- In the process of helping, it should be observed that the client is as active as the worker since the formers participation in the treatment is very necessary. The client should be helped to help himself.
- The worker has also to look to the interest of the family, community and the agency and as such he has to help the client to adjust with the family and the community by releasing the immediate resources available in the community, taking the family as a primary institution. The worker has to consider the client as part of the family, community and society with mutual responsibility.
- In order to establish rapport with the client, the worker should be sincere and sympathetic towards him and sensitive to the clients "feelings and problems".

The Casework Approach

Casework is when you are involved individually with a client who has a problem. It involves interaction between you and your client or a family unit. Casework incorporates the following methods:

a) **Problem-Solving**. The emphasis is on releasing the client's fears and anxieties and motivating him to deal with his problems.

Example: A worried student who has failed to join the course of his/her choice but has other alternatives.

b) **Functional Casework.** This puts emphasis on giving and receiving help. It is built on the basis that human beings use human relationships, including the relationship with you, to find and strengthen their own purpose, and move towards its realization.

Example: A student who wants to join an institution on which she has no information.

c) **Crisis-Oriented Short-Term Casework.** This realizes the vulnerability of individuals in dealing with a personal crisis. Its primary value lies in helping the client deal with his/her emotional upset. In this case, the brevity of the social worker's service, and evidence of its effectiveness are important.

Example: Helping someone who has lost a relative, especially if the death was sudden.

d) **Task-Centered Casework.** This method incorporates crisis intervention, problem solving, and functional approaches. It involves identifying the problem, sharing the task of problemsolving with the client, and setting a deadline for achieving the goals.

Example: A student who is a good athlete but is fearful of competition. You will counsel him, and the trainer will give him more training.

People in these communities are often exposed to considerable stress due to poverty and financial strain, weather, natural disasters, farm crises, and other conditions outside their control. Clients in these communities' experience mood and anxiety disorders; trauma; and cognitive, developmental, and psychotic disorders at rates as least as high as residents of urban areas (Roberts et al. 1999). Suicide rates in rural areas are higher than in urban areas and rural areas have high rates of chronic illness, alcohol abuse, and disability (Roberts et al. 1999; Wagenfeld and Ozarin, D 1988).

Sterling (2009) pointed out the need for workers to educate themselves about local politics, familial history, and local power structures. Workers also need to understand that people living in rural small communities believed that the confidentiality would be broken by workers and thus are reluctant to seek care. It is of utmost importance to maintain the confidentiality of the clients and build trust within these small knit communities. Failure to properly secure and protect confidential business of your client can lead loss of the client via violence or suicide. Client information in the wrong hands is a definite breach of the dyadic relationship and should be a priority for the worker and the agency.

Overall these principles (e.g., individualization, acceptance, self- determination and confidentiality) are conveyed through the use of techniques, assessment tools

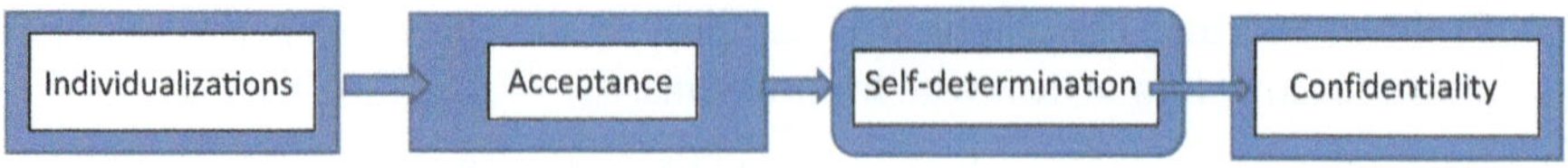

Diagram 3.1 Principles of casework method

and problem-solving skills. The principles of casework method are practicable by means of these techniques (Diagram 3.1).

Review Questions
1. What are the principles of casework method?
2. Name a few of the key contributors to defining the casework method.
3. What does social work method mean?

References

Bosanquet, H. (1914). *Social work in London, 1869–1912: A history of the charity organization society*. New York: E P Button & Co.

Hargrove (1986). Ethical Issues in rural mental health. *Professional Psychology: Research and Practice, 17*(1), 20–23.

Helbok, C. (2010). The practice of psychology in rural communities: Potential ethical dilemmas. *Ethics & Behavior, 13*(4), 367–384.

Hollis, F., & Wood, M. (1981). *Casework: A psychosocial therapy* (3rd ed.). New York: Random House.

National Association of Social Worker Foundation. (2004). NASW social work pioneers. http://www.naswfoundation.org/pioneers/.

Richmond, M. (1917). *Social diagnosis* (Vol. 17, p. 1143). New York: Russell Sage Foundation.

Roberts, L. W., Battaglia, J., & Epstein, R. S. (1999). Frontier ethics: Mental health care needs and ethnical dilemmas in rural communities. *Psychiatric Services, 50*, 497–503. https://doi.org/10.1176/ps.50.4.497.

Sterling, D. (2009). Practicing rural psychotherapy: Complexity of role and boundary. *Journal of Psychotherapy in Private Practice, 10*(3), 105–127.

Urdang, E. (2010). Awareness of self: A critical tool. *Social Work Education: The International Journal, 29*(5), 523–538.

Chapter 4
Theoretical Frameworks of the Social Casework Method

Important Highlights:

- An overview of the Freud Structural Theory.
- An understanding of common defense mechanisms.
- A provided outline of Erikson's Stages of psychosocial development.
- An overview of the Maslow Hierarchy of Needs.
- A comprehensive understanding of family systems.
- A definition of Bronfenbrenner's Ecological Systems Theory.

Historical Philosophical Underpinning of the Social Casework Method

The philosophical assumptions of casework method were developed out of collective thinking of prominent psychologists, social workers, and sociologists in response to fundamental questions; What is the worth and dignity of humans? What is the quality of life? and Is it society's responsibility to find a purpose for humans in life? Every individual reacts differently to social, economic and physical environments, therefore problems are interpreted differently according to the person. The philosophy's understanding of these questions is: every human has to be considered as a person with dignity and worth. Quality of life is measured by some common human needs such as the need to be met for the growth and development of individuals. Every individual has within themselves the potential for growth and achievement and has a right to the realization of this potential. Another tenet is everyone has the capacity to change and society has an obligation to help those who do not have the means for the realization of their potentials.

E. J. Johnson, C. L. Huggins, *Social Casework Methodology: A Skills Handbook for the Caribbean Human Services Worker*, SpringerBriefs in Social Work,
https://doi.org/10.1007/978-3-030-27319-4_4

These are the core beliefs of the social work profession and it is the motivation for social work and social welfare. Non-acceptance of these values is untenable in social work practice and a career in Human services is not meant for those who reject these values. This chapter outlines theoretical frameworks that are essential to be considered when using the casework method in the Caribbean.

Theoretical Frameworks

Foremost social casework method is a humanistic attempt for helping people who have difficulty in coping with the problems of daily living. Humanistic approach (Benjafield 2010) is viewing the individual as more than just a sum of their parts he or she should be viewed holistically. As well as, a person's behavior is influenced by their surrounding environment. Social relationships are key to the development of a human being. People are aware of their existence, that is, they are conscious of themselves and their surroundings however they may not be aware of how past experiences is connected to their present behavior which may have a negative impact on the person. Human beings have *free will* and make *conscious choices*. They are not driven by instinct or impulse alone. Human beings have intentional goals and seek to create meaning in life. Freud's Structural theory clearly explains how humans are emotionally driven.

Freud's Structural Theory

Sigmund Freud's structural theory emerged in the 1920s and it had a strong impact on casework. The new psychoanalytical knowledge pertaining to human behavior was eagerly absorbed by caseworkers which were found useful in understanding clients and their problems. During this period of development, caseworkers focused their attention on psychic forces within the individual. In Freud's seminal book (1933) The Ego and the Id, Freud believed in psychic determinism, in the power of the unconscious mind and in the strength of the instincts. In his view, nothing occurred by chance; all behavior was motivated by unconscious conflicts stemming from early childhood and centering on the expression of aggressive and sexual instincts.

The incidents that occurred during childhood have a definite impact on personality development. Children for example, who experience a lack of love which is a result of being neglected or abused where caretakers do not perform the essential duties of parenting or inflict physical abuse on the children. In some families' severe child-rearing practices such as the parent's inclination to be unduly strict and punishing towards their children may lead a child to inappropriate bonding with the parent. The probable result is that the child will begin to fear their parents more than love them. A fear-based relationship is hostile to growth. Children who experience over-protection where parents overprotect children and are unable to apply discretion or provide limits or checks to children's behavior has an impact on children's personality development. Effective parenting means having a consistent pattern of rearing children. Children learn appropriate ways of behavior and thus parents become models for children's learning. Parents who have inadequate parents or have a defective ego and superego functioning are poor models for their children.

A person's childhood has a significant impact on their personality. A personality is the overall picture of the characteristic behavior of the individual. Behavior includes thinking, feeling, speaking and doing. To understand a person's personality means to inform oneself about the usual way the individual thinks feels, speaks and does things.

Freud identified the psychosexual stages (e.g., oral, anal, phallic and, oedipal) as central in the origination of anxiety, conflicts, defenses, adult character traits and neurotic symptoms. Freud's Structural theory described the ego as one of three structures of the mental apparatus of the personality along with the id (i.e., the seat of instincts) and the superego (i.e., the conscience and the ego-ideal).

The id is the most primitive part of the personality the part that is shared with animals. It is the seat of instincts and is said to operate on the pleasure principle or the principle of instant gratification. Fulfillment of biological needs is the main concern of the id. When a person is hungry the id is activated in the sense that it is driven to make efforts to get food. The ego and superego evolved during the process of human civilization as the human being gradually progressed from the level of a primitive savage. The superego constitutes the individual's values, moral codes, and considerations of what is right and wrong. The ego maintains the balance between the id and the superego in relation to the demands of the environment. When a person is hungry he/she satisfies their hunger through socially approved ways and not through say stealing food. That food should not be stolen comes as a behavioral check from the superego.

The ego is influenced in this context by the prohibitions preceding from the superego as well as the consideration of reality. The ego has various functions: impulse control, tolerance of frustration, postponement of gratification, tension management, reality testing, object relations, and integration and synthesis. Impulse control refers to the function of controlling the id impulses in relation to reality.

The ego controls impulses for immediate satisfaction of these needs and directs the individual to socially approved channels. Tolerance of frustration and postponement of gratification are operative in human life in the day to day living. For example, a child who gives up learning in the face of frustrations of learning and looks for immediate satisfaction will not get educated. The great human achievements would not have been possible had it not been for the effective performance of these functions. The achievers were those people who instead of getting crushed under frustrations preceded ahead with their efforts for attaining their goals by trying new strategies of problem-solving when the old strategies failed and did not deviate from their long-term goals for immediate satisfaction. Understandable the ego is said to operate on the reality principle. The ego by its functions: mediating between the drives (id) and external reality; moderating conflict between drives (id) and the internalized prohibitions against their expression (superego); instituting mechanism (defenses) to protect the ego from the painful experience of anxiety; and playing a crucial role in development through its capacity for identification with external objects. Freud's Structural theory permitted a greater understanding of the individual's negotiations with the external world as well as their personality and the impact of the environment and interpersonal relationships on behavior.

In Freud's (1926) Inhibitions, Symptoms and Anxiety, Freud proposed that defenses arise to mediate between the pressures of instincts and those of the internalized values and prohibitions of the superego. When conflict develops between the id and superego, anxiety emerges and acts as a signal to the ego to institute some type of action to eliminate the anxiety emerges and acts as a signal to the ego to institute some type of action to eliminate the anxiety. Defenses are part of the ego's repertoire of mechanisms for protecting the individual from such anxiety by keeping the intolerable or unacceptable impulses or threats from conscious awareness. Defense mechanisms operate unconsciously. All people use defenses but their exact type and extent vary from individual to individual. Generally given a person favors some defenses over others. Better functioning individuals tend to use defenses flexibly and selectively rather than rigidly and pervasively. All defense mechanisms falsify or distort reality to some extent, although in individuals who function more effectively such distortions are minimal or transient and do not impair the person's ability to test reality. Defenses enable the person to function optimally without undue anxiety they are said to be effective. In many instances, however depending on the intensity of the conflict the nature of the current stimuli evoking it or the fragility or pervasiveness of the defense itself such mechanisms may prove to be ineffective and maladaptive. They may prevent the individual from gaining needed satisfaction; be insufficient to contain the anxiety or conflict so that the person becomes overwhelmed, symptomatic or disorganized; distort reality to such a degree that overall ego functioning is impaired.

Common Defense Mechanisms

Common defense mechanisms were identified by Anna Freud, Sigmund Freud's last child. She identified nine mechanisms that were commonly used to hide anxiety and distort reality (Freud 1936). The following are basic defense mechanisms used infrequently.

Denial- involves a negation or non-acceptance of important aspects of reality or of one's own experience of important aspects or reality or of one's own experience that one may perceive. A person may refuse to recognize they have diabetes because assimilation of this knowledge is too traumatic so they refuse to take medication and change their diet.

Somatization- is intolerable impulses or conflicts are converted into physical symptoms. A woman who recently suffered a break up will become very ill and lose a lot of weight and think is has cancer.

Repression- a high-level defense involved keeping unwanted thoughts and feelings out of awareness or unconscious. Repression may involve loss of memory for specific incidents, especially traumatic events. A young woman is told repeatedly that her mother is dead when she was 10 years old. Despite her love for her mother, her presence at the time of the event she has no conscious recall of the incident.

Isolation- A form of repression of the feelings associated with a particular content of the ideas connected with certain effects. The is accompanied by experiencing feelings in relation to a different situation. A young man is unable to be in touch with sad feelings when discussing a traumatic event but will cry bitterly when viewing a TV commercial.

Projection- when the individual attributes to others unacceptable thought and feelings that the person has but that are not conscious this is projection. It involves serious distortions of others' feelings, attitudes, and behavior. A person has a strong desire for something but says that his friend wants the object even more.

Undoing- this defense is termed the 'psychological erasure in that involves nullifying or voiding symbolically an unacceptable or guilt-provoking act, thought or feeling. A man is very attracted to his secretary so he may buy his wife an expensive gift.

Regression- this involves the return to an earlier developmental phase, level of functioning, or type of behavior in order to avoid the anxieties of the present. Behaviors that have been given up recurs. A man who gave up smoking 20 years ago recently suffered a significant loss in his business and started smoking again.

Sublimation- it is converting an impulse from a socially objectionable aim to a socially acceptable one while still retaining the original goal of the impulse. A man who has fantasies of having sex with children will have a sexual relationship with an adult while still fantasizing about children.

Reaction Formation- involves keeping certain impulses out of awareness by replacing the impulse in consciousness with its opposite. A husband who censors his unacceptable angry feelings toward his wife may act in a particularly loving way when irritated by her.

These are a few yet pertinent defense mechanisms and it operates outside conscious awareness, it is not a deliberate attempt to work through a problem with these mechanisms. These mechanisms work to mediate the id, ego and the superego and it is often times unconscious. It is different from coping mechanisms which are conscious and purposeful. The difference between defense and coping mechanisms is defense mechanisms are rigid, compelled, channeled and perhaps conditioned and coping mechanisms are flexible, purposive and is used by choice. Defense mechanisms distort the present situation rather than being oriented to reality requirements of the present situation. Defenses operate as if it were necessary and possible wholly to remove disturbing effects and may involve magical thinking rather than operate in accordance with reality.

It is crucial to undertake a full evaluation of a person's ego function before undertaking any type of counseling or intervention in order to understand their defense versus their coping mechanisms.

Erikson's Stages of Psychosocial Development

Erikson's theory provides a rationale for therapeutic approaches that address the dynamic interplay between current life cycle needs and the inner and other resources available to meet them and that involve interventions directed beyond the individual psyche. In Erik Erikson's important books Childhood and Society (1950) and Identity and the Life Cycle (1959) Erikson proposed that the human life cycle from birth to death could be conceived of a series of eight successive stages. Erikson highlighted the interplay of instinctual and psychosocial factors in ego development. It is an individual's need to adapt the physiological and psychological needs and capacities to the expectations, challenges and opportunities, constraints and resources of the social environment. Erikson described each stage of the life cycle as having a core psychosocial crisis, the resolution is essential to optimal healthy functioning. The term 'crisis' reflects the idea that there is a state of tension at the beginning of each new stage.

Each psychosocial crisis described by Erikson is briefly described.

Basic trust v. Basic Mistrust – an infant must develop a sense of basic conviction in the predictability of the world and its fulfillment of the person's needs.

Autonomy v. Shame and Doubt- In the second year of life, the infant seeks to be independent and autonomous while at the same time the infant is pulled by his dependency needs.

Initiative v. Guilt- Once the child develops some form of autonomy over themselves and in the interaction with the environment the child is ready to broaden his horizons. The child moves to become a particular kind of person that he or she wants to be. The development of gender identification, appropriate sex-role behavior and conscience are important in this phase. Sexual curiosity is intense.

Industry v. Inferiority- In this stage, the child develops a sense that he can be useful and produce things the child learns to persevere and complete tasks.

Identity v. Role Confusion- During adolescence continue to develop their identity and this stage is the tension between integrating one's past, present and future and it also entails the integration of past identifications with others into a whole that represents one's unique self. The role confusion often may adopt dysfunctional or antisocial behavior as a way of achieving some type of identity, even a negative one.

Intimacy v. Distantiation and Self-absorption- Young adulthood is about intimate relationships with others to achieve intimacy or isolation or self-absorption.

Generativity v. Stagnation- Generativity is carrying out the responsibility for the next generation by supporting others and the society in areas relating to the promotion of values versus not contributing to society at all.

Integrity v. Despair and Disgust. It implies an emotional integration and acceptance of all of one's past experiences and brings a readiness to face death (Diagram 4.1).

Erikson's theories paved the way of primary prevention through interventions aimed at improving adaptive fits between caretakers and children as well as between individuals and environmental resources. During the 1930s during the economic

Diagram 4.1 Maslow hierarchy of needs

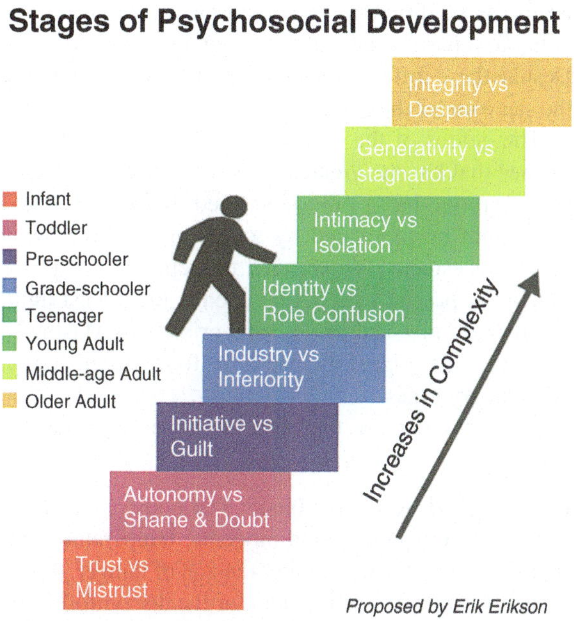

depression workers utilizing the casework, the method had to consider the economic factors as a cause of the distress of clients. There was also the realization that economic distress could lead to emotional distress and breakdown. Caseworkers had to consider environmental factors that may impact a client's functioning. Freud's structural theory is just one of many theories to explain personality development. Erikson stages of psychosocial development provide a clear definition of the psychosocial influences during the life cycle

Abraham Maslow (1908–1970) sought to understand the conditions needed for human beings to reach their fullest potential. He felt that people are basically trustworthy, self- protecting, and self-governing and have an innate tendency toward growth and are even capable of love but the conditions have to be available to reach these goals. According to Maslow's theory, there are four types of needs that must be satisfied before a person can act unselfishly. The needs are arranged in a hierarchical order and the upward climb is made by satisfying one set of needs at a time. The most basic drives are physiological. After that comes the need for safety, then the desire for love, and then the quest for esteem. We're driven to satisfy the lower needs, but we're drawn to meet the higher ones. Maslow referred to the four lower needs as "deficiency needs" because their lack creates a tension within us. As long as we can work to satisfy the cravings, we're moving toward growth. Satisfying needs is healthy. Blocking gratification makes us sick. The urge to fulfill needs is potent but not overpowering.

People can resist the pull of physiological, safety, love, and esteem needs, but it's not easy. Although everyone has the same set of needs, our ways of fulfilling those needs can be different. You could meet your need to belong (love and be loved) by going to a party, whereas your roommate might go for a quiet walk with a friend. Despite these different means of gratification, our common desire for love makes us the same under the skin.

The genius of the hierarchy is its concept of prepotency. A prepotent need is the one that has the greatest power or influence over our actions. Maslow claimed that everyone has a prepotent need, but the need will differ among individuals. You might be motivated by a craving for love, while I may be motivated by a desire for esteem. Which need is prepotent for a given individual? According to Maslow, a person's prepotent need is the lowest unmet need in the pyramid. Not surprisingly physical drives take priority in Maslow's system. Almost all motivational theorists regard the needs for food and other physical necessities as powerful and primary urges.

The following are the hierarchy of needs from the lowest drive to the highest (Maslow 1943) (Diagram 4.2).

Physiological needs are basic The body craves food, liquid, sleep, oxygen, sex, freedom of movement, and moderate temperature. When any of these are in short supply, we feel the distressing tension of hunger, thirst, fatigue, shortness of breath, sexual frustration, confinement, or the discomfort of being too hot or cold.

The safety needs operate mainly on a psychological level. Naturally, we try to avoid a poke in the eye with a sharp stick. But once we've managed a certain level of physical comfort, we'll seek to establish stability and consistency in a

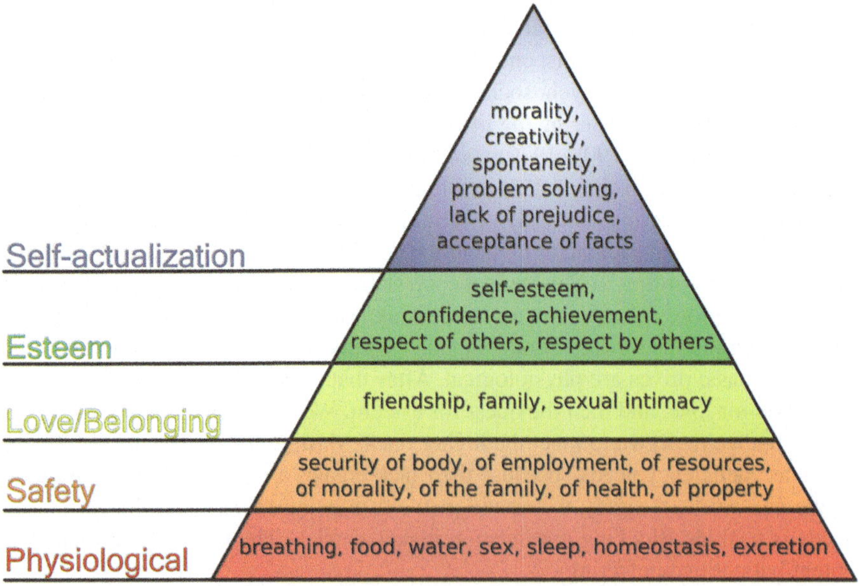

Diagram 4.2 Hierarchy of needs from the lowest drive to the highest

chaotic world. When he talked about security. Maslow also placed religious inclination on the safety rung because he saw that tendency as an attempt to bring about an ordered universe.

The love or belongingness needs come into play after the physiological and security drives are satisfied. Gratification is a matter of degree rather than an either-accomplishment. But once a need has been significantly satisfied over a long period of time, it becomes functionally absent. The action switches to the next highest level, in this case, love. Maslow's concept of belonging combines the twin urges to give and receive love. For Maslow, giving love is seeking to fill a void by understanding and accepting selected others. Receiving love is a way of staving off the pangs of loneliness and rejection. Even though it's higher in the hierarchy than physical or safety needs, the desire for love and belonging is similar in that it motivates only when a person feels a deficit.

The esteem needs are of two types. There's self-esteem, which is the result of competence or mastery of tasks. This "need for achievement." There's also the attention and recognition that come from others. Wanting this admiration is part of the "need for power." The individual differences in needs are tied to personality, and they change slowly if at all. Maslow, on the other hand, believes that repeated shifts in motivation are possible when a person is in a supportive environment.

Maslow described the need for **self-actualization** as "the desire to become more and more what one is, to become everything that one is capable of becoming". People feel this gentle but persistent tug to maximize their potential only after they have satisfied their basic deficiency cravings. Maslow's hierarchy of needs is a pivotal theory that operationalizes an individual's instincts and the motivational factors for behavior change and the internal factors that impact clients.

In the twentieth century, the development of systems theory had a tremendous effect on the way scientist and researcher in the biological, and social sciences understood the way environment from the natural ecosystems to the human family function.

Systems Theory

Systems theory provides a conceptual perspective that can guide the interactions of various systems in the environment including individuals, groups, families, organizations, and communities (Braziller 1976). A system is a set of elements that are interrelated to make a functional whole. A person, a family, a church, a school, and the community are all systems. Each with many components that work together in order to function as long as all elements have some relationship to each other and arranged in some pattern that is interrelated and function as a whole is not simply random. Elements a system must have some kind of mutual relationship or connection with each other and must be functional. Together, they must be able to perform some regular task, activity, or function and fulfill some purpose.

A client system is any individual, family, group, organization, or community that will ultimately benefit from an intervention. Individuals, families, organization, and communities are considered a client system. The target of change has to be specified and understood to create and implement an action system. An action system undertakes the planned change process to change an agency policy, develop a new program or institute some project such as evaluating intervention methodology. This action system will be discussed in the casework process section.

The Family System

The family system and dynamics is also a branch of systems that is important for social service workers to know and doing casework. A family is defined as a group of people who love each other (Seligman and Darling 2007). It is important to understand every client even if they are living alone originally grew up in a complex family system that has profoundly on his or her environment. The family system represents a subsystem of the larger community of which the following assumptions are made (Seligman and Darling 2007).

1. *Changing one part of the system will lead to changes in other parts of the system.*
2. *Families are always changing over the life span, family members assume different roles.*
3. *Families are generally open systems in that they receive information and exchange it with each other and with people outside the family. Families vary in their degree of openness (e.g., allowing people into the family) and closedness (e.g., not allowing people in the family), which can vary over time and according to circumstances. Family systems are open or closed depending on the degree to which that are organized and interact with the outside environment. Closed systems are rarely if ever, completely isolated or closed off from the outside. For a family to be truly operating in a closed system, all outside transactions and communications would have to cease to exist, which is highly improbable.*
4. *Individual dysfunction is often reflective of an active emotional system.*

The composition of the family has several manifestations which encompass many different patterns. The family consists of four major subsystems, including (1) spousal in the broadest sense; (2) parent-child; (3) sibling; (4) the smallest subsystem, the individual. Each family member also engages in different roles within a family system that can change depending on the family dynamics and external circumstances. Roles are defined as 'actual patterns of interaction with others.'

Different family compositions includes the nuclear family, a family that encompasses only parents and unmarried children; single-parent families, a family consisting of one parent and children; a common-in-law union, a family including two adults in a relationship but are not legally married with or without children; a reconstituted family consisting of a husband or wife with children from a previous marriage/union of one of the spouses; a blended family consisting of a husband and wife who are not necessarily married that includes children from one or more marriages/unions; an extended family, which includes more than parents and unmarried children but also grandparents, married children or other relatives living in the same residence; a consanguine family, consisting of a family in which the primary emphasis is on the blood relationship of parents and children or brothers and sisters rather on the marital relationships of husband/ wife relationship.

In the Caribbean, family compositions were created due to its historical background of slavery and the colonization of the Caribbean islands. There was a lot of sexual relations between the races and between the slaves and slave owners. There was a lot of nocturnal rambles and multiple mistresses (Chamberlain 2006). Until the eighteenth century, slave marriages were neither promoted nor recognized. Slave families were also discarded. At the end of the eighteenth century, Christian marriage began to be encouraged on plantations as a way to improve fertility and to deflect criticism from abolitionists. Christian marriage, when it occurred was accepted not as the prerequisite to family formation but its opposite as a confirmation and celebration of a couple's loyalty and fertility (Chamberlain 2006). Marriage followed a particular pattern as younger slaves enjoyed what is now termed visiting relations, with their partner, from whom children may or may not have resulted. While these visiting relations did not involve co-habituating they were considered a serious relationship. The second phase was that of cohabitation practiced by older slaves and often leading to the final stage of marriage.

In the Caribbean, the practice of accepting friends as kin is common in the Caribbean and it was initiated during the middle passage as an attempt to civilize the impact of slavery and to form of attachment for people who were on the same vessel from Africa. Kinship relations was a form of social behavior. It is customary for persons who were older to be called 'Uncle', 'Aunty', 'Tatta', 'Mama', sister between people who had no obvious blood relations (Chamberlain 2006). There was also an African understanding of family which includes polygamy, a man with two or more wives. The legacy of slavery and the dismantling of the African family, the dominance of Christianity in the culture, which promotes marriage as a primary way to form a family as well as the environmental circumstances of living in the Caribbean which can be rural and farm like communities (Barrow 2000). The following are different forms of families that typically live together in the Caribbean:

Marital families, simple family or primary family- the parents are married with or without their children and possibly adopted children and non-kin persons living in the household.

Secondary families- which is of the unmarried adult, lives outside the home but has children for a person who is married to someone else.

Disintegrate families- households containing women, children and grandchildren with no male figures.

Extended families- which is the marital families and children live with other kin (e.g., grandparents)

Faithful concubinage- unmarried domestic partners living together.

Sibling households- where the adults residents are all siblings living along with their children.

Companionate unions- cohabiting unions of less than 3 years duration.

Systems and especially family systems are important for the casework process because it provides a description of the client's environment and can highlight areas that need to be more strengthened and supported.

Bronfenbrenner's Ecological Systems Theory

The development and socialization of individuals are influenced by the different circles of the environment with which a person has in active inter-relationship. This includes three significant assumptions: (1) person is an active player, exerting influence on his/her environment, (2) the environment is compelling the person to adapt to its conditions and restrictions and (3) environment is understood to consist of different size entities that are placed one inside another, of their reciprocal relationships and of micro-, meso-, exo- and macrosystems. (Bronfenbrenner 1977). Bronfenbrenner (1989) ecological systems theory identified four levels of social systems that make up the social context of human development (Diagram 4.3).

The microsystem is comprised of a person's relationships in his or her immediate settings (e.g., family, school, church). Individuals belong to multiple microsystems (e.g., family, school, sports team). The mesosystem refers to interrelationships

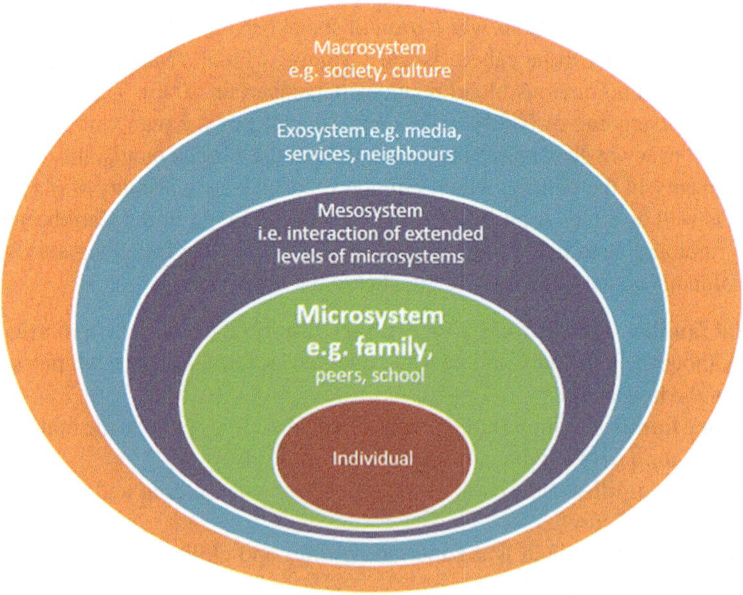

Diagram 4.3 Ecological systems theory

between or among microsystems. The mesosystem comprises of linkages and processes taking place between two or more settings containing the client (e.g., the relations between home and school, school and workplace etc.). In other words, a mesosystem is a system of microsystems. The exo-system refers to larger social systems that the individual does not participate indirectly, but that influence his or her life (e.g., government). The exosystem, encompasses the linkage and processes taking place between two or more settings, at least one of which does not ordinarily contain the developing person, but in which events occur that influence processes within the immediate settings that does contain that person (e.g. for a child, relation between the home and the parent's workplace).

Finally, the macro-system refers to the broader cultural context in which all the other systems are located. The macrosystem consists of the overarching pattern of micro-, meso-, and exosystems characteristic of a given culture, subculture, or other broader social context such as, systems, resources, lifestyles, life course options, and patterns of social interchange that are embedded in each of these systems. The macrosystem can be thought of as a societal blueprint for a particular culture, subculture, or other broader social contexts. Last, the chronosystem is a description of the evolution, development or stream of development of the external systems in time. The chronosystem models can cover either a short or long period of time (Bronfenbrenner 1989).

There are some similarities that exist between systems theory and ecological theory. Both emphasize systems and focus on the dynamic interaction among many systems. Some of the terms and mechanisms are similar. Additionally, each provides human service workers with a framework with which to view the world. Finally, both perspectives emphasize external interactions and how helping people improve their interactions with other systems.

These were just a few of the theories in the development of the casework method. Freud's structural theory is just one of many theories to explain personality development. Erikson stages of psychosocial development provide a clear definition of the psychosocial influences on the life cycle and Maslow Hierarchy of needs describes the physiological needs that humans need to survive. Last systems theory, family systems, Bronfenbrenner's Ecological Systems Theory provides a clear depiction of how environment, society and the community interplay and impact the individual and the family.

Person-Centered Approach

The Person-Centered Approach developed from the work of the psychologist Dr. Carl Rogers (1902–1987). He advanced an approach to psychotherapy and counselling that, at the time (the1940s – 1960s), was considered extremely radical if not revolutionary.

Originally described as non-directive, this therapy moved away from the idea that the therapist was the expert and towards a theory that trusted the innate

Diagram 4.4 Person-centered approach

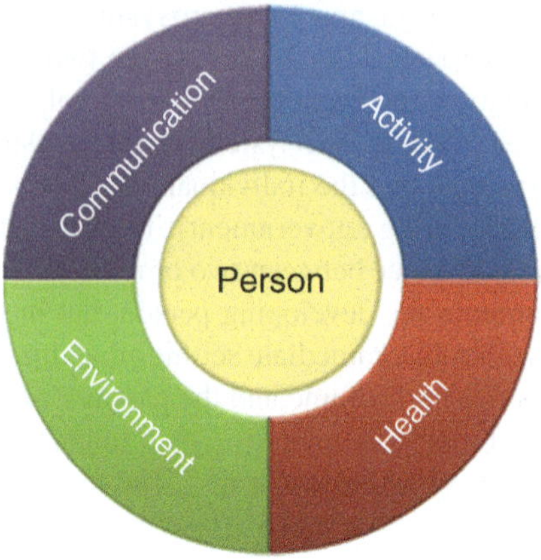

tendency (known as the actualizing tendency) of human beings to find fulfillment of their personal potentials. An important part of this theory is that in a particular psychological environment, the fulfillment of personal potentials includes sociability, the need to be with other human beings and a desire to know and be known by other people. It also includes being open to experience, being trusting and trustworthy, being curious about the world, being creative and compassionate.

The psychological environment described by Rogers was one where a person felt free from threat, both physically and psychologically. This environment could be achieved when being in a relationship with a person who was deeply understanding (empathic), accepting (having unconditional positive regard) and genuine (congruent) (Diagram 4.4).

Although initially developed as an approach to psychotherapy (eventually becoming known as client/person-centered therapy/counseling), Rogers and his colleagues came to believe that their ideas could be transferred to other areas where people were in relationships. For example, teaching, management, childcare, patient care, conflict resolution.

Today there are many people who, although not working as psychotherapists and counselors, use the work of Rogers as guiding principles in their day-to-day work and relationships. At one level, Rogers' theory and work are very simple to describe. As many people would attest, both those using the approach and those working as person-therapists/counselors, it can be very difficult to put into practice because the approach does not use techniques but relies on the personal qualities of the therapist/person to build a non-judgemental and empathic relationship.

Review Questions

1. What do you see at the greatest challenge you would face when working with families in the Caribbean?
2. Name a theoretical framework that you believe is most effective when working with clients.
3. Which theoretical framework do you think is relevant when working with multiple systems?

References

Barrow. (2000). *Family in the Caribbean*. Jamaica: Ian Randle Publishers.
Benjafield, J. (2010). The golden section and American Psychology 1892–1938. *Journal of the History of the Behavior Science, 46*(1), 52–71.
Braziller, G. (1976). *General system theory: Foundations, development, applications*. New York: George Braziller Inc.
Bronfenbrenner, U. (1977). Toward an experimental ecology of human development. *American Psychologist, 32*(7), 513–531. https://doi.org/10.1037/0003-066X.32.7.513.
Bronfenbrenner, U. 1989. Ecological systems theory. *Annals of Child Development. 6*, 187–249.
Chamberlain, M. (2006). *Migration and the Anglo-Caribbean experience family love in the Diaspora*. Jamaica: Ian Randle Publishers.
Erikson, E. (1950). *Childhood and society*. New York: W.W. Norton Books.
Erikson, E. (1959). Identity and the life cycle. *Psychological Issues, 1*, 50–100.
Freud, S. (1926). *Inhibitions, symptoms, and anxiety.*. In the Standard Edition (Vol. 20). London: Hogarth Press.
Freud, S. (1933). Anxiety and the instinctual life. In *New introductory lectures in psychoanalysis*. The Standard Edition (Vol. 23). London: Hogarth Press.
Freud, A. (1936). *The ego and the mechanisms of defense*. New York: International Universities Press.
Maslow, A.H. (1943). A theory of human motivation. Psychological Review, 50(4), 370–396. https://doi.org/10.1037/h0054346–viapsychclassics.yorku.ca.
Seligman, M., & Darling, R. (2007). *Ordinary families, special children: A systems approach to childhood disability* (3rd ed.). New York: Guilford Publications.

Chapter 5
Theoretical Underpinnings Needed for the Caribbean

Important Highlights:

- An overview of intersectionality.
- Define resiliency theory.
- An understanding of cultural humility.

Anti-Oppressive Practice

Anti-oppressive practice is a form of radical theory in social work practice. Radical practice (Fook 1993) is concerned about the potential for casework to not pathologize the individual and make all the problems the client is facing all their fault. Its focus is to ensure casework is informed by understanding the barriers caused by social status, race, ethnicity, religion, inequality. The common themes of radical social work are: an analysis that a client's personal problems can be traced to the causes in the socio-economic structure, therefore the individual is a 'victim' of these problematic social structures and the client should not be blamed for causing the problem. There should be an on-going critique of the existing social, political and economic arrangements that impact clients. There should be an on-going analysis of the social control functions of the social work profession and the social welfare system. There should be a commitment to protecting the individual person against oppression by more powerful individuals, groups and structures. Lastly, there should be goals of powerful liberation and social change. In order to reduce poverty, helping families strive towards social and structural change. It is meant to challenge the status quo and to provide radical ideas by sharing experiences, discussing current events, clarifying views and developing an awareness of social issues.

As social service workers working in the Caribbean there should be a critical consciousness," Friere (1972) focuses on challenging individual assumptions,

E. J. Johnson, C. L. Huggins, *Social Casework Methodology: A Skills Handbook for the Caribbean Human Services Worker*, SpringerBriefs in Social Work,
https://doi.org/10.1007/978-3-030-27319-4_5

aiding the client, and advocating for and creating change within society. The critical consciousness must analyze current structural institutions (e.g. education) to identify power imbalances as a social service worker assist that actions that could be taken to dismantle oppressive structures for clients. There should be an awareness of differences and open-mindedness which is necessary to understand a client's situation. The social service worker must be broad enough to account for a client who is of the LGBTI community and understand the client's history and the structural factors that maintain oppression. For the social service worker practicing the casework method, it is important to engage in the fight against social injustice as they are working directly with their clients. Workers should strive to question the status quo and analyze current agency and societal structures. Some theories that should be integrated into the theoretical underpinning of the casework method in the Caribbean such as, resiliency theory, intersectionality, and cultural humility.

Resiliency

An anti-oppressive social work framework that should be considered in the casework method for the Caribbean client in the resiliency theory. The concept of resilience was developed to relative resistance to psychosocial risk experiences that may otherwise psychological impact the pact (Rutter 2012). It has been defined as a dynamic process having a positive adaptation within the context of significant adversity (Luthar et al. 2003). Resilience is the process of coping with adversity, change, or opportunity in a manner that results in the identification, fortification, and enrichment of resilient qualities or protective factors. Resiliency is conceptualized as relative resistance to stressors or adversity. The central constructs of the theory included risk factors/mechanisms, vulnerability factors, and protective factors/mechanisms (Diagram 5.1).

Risk factors have been conceptualized either as (1) the adverse events or conditions (for example, poverty) that can for which there is empirical place duress on a person which can cause psychopathology, illness, or dysfunctional developmental outcomes or as (2) factors that operate to reduce resistance to stressors/adversity.

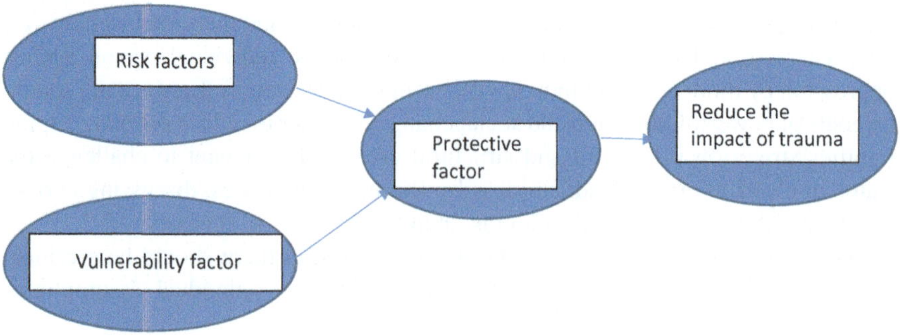

Diagram 5.1 Resiliency process

Vulnerability factors are traits, genetic predispositions, or environmental and biological deficits (such as cognitive impairments) for which there is empirical evidence of heightened response, sensitivity, or reaction to stressors or risk factors. The constructs of vulnerability factors and risk factors are sometimes used interchangeably. Protective factors and mechanisms are traits, contextual characteristics, and interventions that operate to enhance or promote resistance, or which may moderate the effect of the impact of risk factors and functional developmental outcomes. Rutter (2012) suggests that protective mechanisms may operate in one of four ways which are to allow overcoming odds in the face of adversity: by reducing risk impact, by reducing negative chain reactions to risk factors, by promoting resiliency traits (i.e., the opposite of vulnerability factors, such as self-efficacy and optimism), and by setting up new opportunities for success. Reducing risk impact can occur not only by way of buffering events and social networks but also by inoculation due to successful coping with earlier, milder stressful events. Protective and risk mechanisms have been found to vary according to the type of adversity, type of resilient outcome, and life stage under analysis; risk factors in one context may be protective in another (Rutter 2012; Smith-Osborne 2007; Ungar 2004)

Intersectionality

In the 1989 landmark essay "Demarginalizing the Intersection of Race and Sex: A Black Feminist Critique of Anti-discrimination Doctrine, Feminist Theory and Anti-racist Politics," Kimberlé Crenshaw introduced the term to address the marginalization of Black women within not only anti-discrimination law but also in feminist and antiracist theory and politics in the United States, this concept also pertains to the Caribbean (Crenshaw 1991). Intersectionality highlights the ways in which social movement organization and advocacy around violence against women elided the vulnerabilities of black women, particularly women living in poverty.

Intersectionality is the idea that multiple identities intersect to create a whole that is different from the component identities. For example, if you are male, black, and educated, you will be treated differently and in a more oppressive way then if you are white, male and educated. These identities that can intersect include gender, race, social class, ethnicity, nationality, sexual orientation, religion, age, mental disability, physical disability, mental illness, and physical illness as well as other forms of identity.

The lived experience that is often constructed by the interaction of multiple identities and statuses. such as gender, sexual orientation, ability status, age, race/ethnicity, socioeconomic status, immigration and acculturation status, place of residence, may exacerbate the effects of the oppression of racism. For example, you will be treated differently if you are, male, gay, 35, white and a physician that if you are male, gay, 35, black and a cashier at a grocery in the Caribbean. Although being gay is not widely accepted in most Caribbean islands, a white educated gay male is insulated from prejudices and assaults, this may not be the case for the black male. It is an idea that social identities such as race, gender, and class interact to form qualitatively different meanings and experiences. This formulation stands in contrast to the conceptualization of social identities as functioning independently and as added together to form an experience. This framework, it is argued, can be used to understand how systemic injustice and social inequality occurs in a multidimensional basis. Intersectionality holds that the classical conceptualizations of oppression within society—such as racism, sexism, classism, ableism, homophobia, transphobia, xenophobia and belief-based bigotry—do not act independently of each other. Instead, these forms of oppression interrelate, creating a system of oppression that reflects the "intersection" of multiple forms of discrimination.

This term captures the idea that social identities stem from group membership and these social identities reinforce and naturalize one another creating both oppression and opportunity for the individual. At a personal level, intersectionality affects the individual's experience of their own social spheres. At the socio-structural level, the individual's legal status resources or social needs may advantage them or marginalize them. Veenstra's (2012) understanding of intersectionality is focusing on perspectives of individuals with multiple subordinate statuses, such as women of color and the quantity of disadvantage they face. The systems of inequality have a multiplicative effect on experiences of oppression and that some oppressed statuses are simply more at risk than others. It is also a matrix of domination in which all identities interact to create stressful life situations (Diagram 5.2).

In the Caribbean on most islands, the color of one's skin tone and hair texture play a substantial role in how people are treated. Colorism, or discrimination based on skin tone, stems from the preference for proximity to whiteness. Colorism is described as, "Prejudice or discrimination against individuals with a dark skin tone, typically among people of the same ethnic or racial group. Colorism is a global phenomenon, which affects communities of color all over the world. However, histories of slavery and colonialism have resulted in the prominence of colorism within diasporic black communities including the Caribbean, where millions of African individuals were shipped during the Atlantic slave trade. The combination of the mixing of the races such as; white and blacks or black and Indians, or blacks and indigenous people, the color of one's skin tone unconsciously determined one's station in life.

Colorism, a term coined by Alice Walker in 1982 is not a synonym for *racism*. Numerous factors can contribute to "race"(including ancestry); therefore, the racial categorization does not solely rely on skin color. Skin color is only one mechanism used to assign individuals to a racial category, but race is the set of beliefs and assumptions assigned to that category. Racism is the dependence of social status on the social meaning attached to race; colorism is the dependence of social status on skin color *alone*. In order for a form of discrimination to be considered colorism, differential treatment must not result from racial categorization, but from the social values associated with skin color. The darker you are and a female the more relegated you are to the back of society by your own family. In the Caribbean, the lighter you are with straighter hair texture the more accepted you are in society.

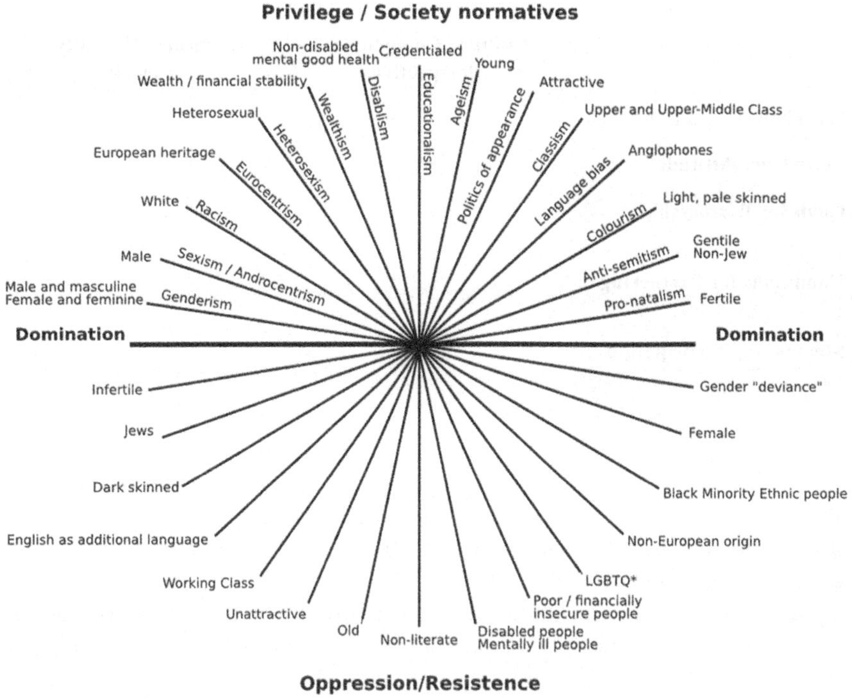

Diagram 5.2 Intersectionality wheel

Cultural Humility

Cultural humility is one construct for understanding and developing a process-oriented approach to competency. Hook et al. (2013) conceptualize cultural humility as the "ability to maintain an interpersonal stance that is other-oriented (or open to the other) in relation to aspects of cultural identity that are most important to the [person]" (p. 2).

When we do not know something, are we able to say that we do not know? Willingness to act on the acknowledgment that we have not and will not arrive at a finish line is integral to this aspect of cultural humility as well. Understanding is only as powerful as the action that follows. There is a difference between cultural competence and cultural humility and it is with cultural competence it makes you the expert in the client's culture something that is to learned and achieved and with cultural humility the social service worker is open, non-judgemental and explorative while allowing the client to be the expert in their own life (Table 5.1).

Three factors guide a sojourner toward cultural humility. The first aspect is a **lifelong commitment to self-evaluation and self-critique** (Tervalon and

Table 5.1 Two perspectives on inclusion and diversity in building partnerships

	Cultural Competence Perspective	Cultural Humility Perspective
Life chances and Long Term Care Attitude		
Goals for Partnership		
Conditions for Partnering		
Meaningful Participation		

Murray-Garcia 1998). Underlying this piece is the knowledge that we are never finished — we never arrive at a point where we are done learning. Therefore, we must be humble and flexible, bold enough to look at ourselves critically and desire to learn more.

The second feature of cultural humility is a desire to **fix power imbalances** where none ought to exist (Tervalon and Murray-Garcia 1998). Recognizing that each person brings something different to the proverbial table of life helps us see the value of each person. When practitioners interview clients, the client is the expert on his or her own life, symptoms and strengths. The practitioner holds a body of knowledge that the client does not like casework skill; however, the client also has an understanding outside the scope of the practitioner. Both people must collaborate and learn from each other for the best outcomes in the client lives. One holds power in scientific knowledge, the other holds power in personal history and preferences.

Finally, cultural humility includes aspiring to **develop partnerships with people and groups who advocate for others** (Tervalon and Murray-Garcia 1998). Though individuals can create positive change, communities and groups can also have a profound impact on systems. We cannot individually commit to self-evaluation and fixing power imbalances without advocating within the larger organizations in which we participate. Cultural humility, by definition, is larger than our individual selves — we must advocate for it systemically.

Multiracial and multi-ethnic individuals and families illustrate the cultural richness of our diverse nation. As therapists, we have a responsibility to recognize and value the diversity of our clients. We must enter our therapeutic relationships with cultural humility, acknowledging that we are always in the process of learning and growing (Diagram 5.3).

Overall, in this chapter, the theoretical framework that should be considered in the Caribbean is to understand the structures of oppression shapes the experience of the vulnerable population such as; resilience, intersectionality, and cultural humility.

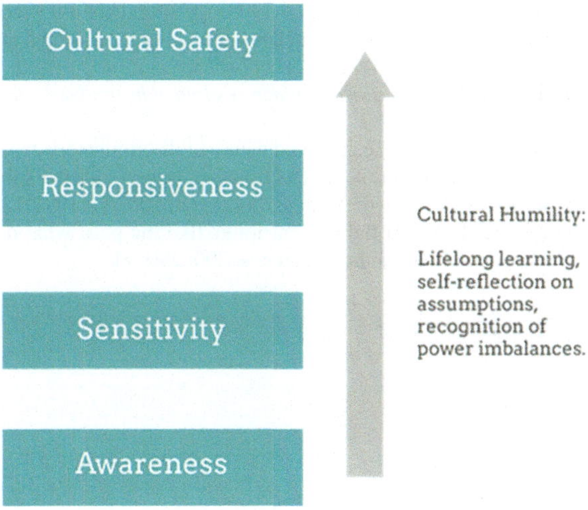

Diagram 5.3 Cultural humility

Review Questions

1. Explain how cultural humility is important for social service workers to work with clients.
2. Demonstrate how intersectionality impacts a dark-skin African woman with no education is impacted in society compared to light-skinned educated women.
3. Explain how risk and protectives factors determine how a person demonstrates resiliency after a traumatic event.

References

Crenshaw, K. (1991). Mapping the margins: Intersectionality, identity politics and violence against women of color. *Stanford Law Review, 43*(3), 1241–1299. http://www.jstor.org/stable/1229039.

Freire, P. (1972). *Pedagogy of the oppressed*. New York: Herder & Herder.

Fook, J. (1993). *Radical casework: A theory of practice*. Australia: Allen & Unwin.

Hook, J. N., Davis, D. E., Owen, J., Worthington, E. L., Jr., & Utsey, S. O. (2013). Cultural humility: Measuring openness to culturally diverse clients. *Journal of Counseling Psychology, 60*, 353–366. https://doi.org/10.1037/a0032595.

Luthar, S. Cicchetti, D., Becker, B. (2003). The construction of Resilience: A critical evaluation and guidelines for future work. *Child Development, 71*, 543–562. https://doi.org/10.1111/1467-8624.00164.

Rutter, M. (2012). Special section article resilience as a dynamic concept. *Development and Psychopathology, 24*(2012), 335–344. # Cambridge University Press. https://doi.org/10.1017/S0954579412000028.

Smith-Osborne, A. (2007). Life span and resiliency theory: A critical review. *Advances in Social Work, 8*(1), 152–168.

Tervalon, M., & Murray-García, J. (1998). Cultural humility versus cultural competence: A critical distinction in defining physician training outcome in multicultural education. *Journal Health Care Poor Underserved, 9*(2), 117–125.

Ungar, M. (2004). *Nurturing hidden resilience in troubled youth*. Toronto: University of Toronto Press.

Veenstra, G. (2012). The gendered nature of discriminatory experiences by race, class, and sexuality: A comparison of intersectionality theory and the subordinate male target hypothesis. *Sex Roles, 68*, 646–659. https://doi.org/10.1007/s11199-012-0243-2.

Walker, A. (1983). If the present looks like the past, what does the future look like? (1982). In Search of our mothers' gardens. 290: 290–91.

Chapter 6
Components of the Social Casework Method

Important Highlights:

- Working with mandated clients.
- Characteristics of the client's personality.
- An overview of the presenting problem.
- The importance of facial expressions.
- The importance of active listening.
- Define empowerment in the casework method.
- The importance of an agency.

The Client vs. Family and Friends

Mandated Client

The mandated client is a person who receives social services either because of a court order or under the threat of some other legal sanction such as the threat of one's children being removed. Even if the client is willing to receive services they can be considered mandated in that they have no real choice to refuse assistance. There are also clients who are also semi mandated because although they not be subjected to mandated assistance and intervention they seek services because they are experiencing some form of external pressure to do so (e.g., family pressure or a threat of police intervention). Similarly, a person with a drug addiction may seek counseling as part of a strategy to provide a court of law with evidence of their commitment to rehabilitation clients who are forced by such concerns cannot be considered truly willing but neither are they mandated clients (De Jong and Berg 2001). Another type of semi-mandated clients is those who are receiving services because they have a practical need for the

E. J. Johnson, C. L. Huggins, *Social Casework Methodology: A Skills Handbook for the Caribbean Human Services Worker*, SpringerBriefs in Social Work,
https://doi.org/10.1007/978-3-030-27319-4_6

services offered by a social service agency. For example, women and children seeking shelter because of domestic violence will also have services available to them. Clients seeking accommodation services may not seek and may actively resist social casework services that are often provided in conjunction with the shelter.

Working with mandated clients can be difficult and sometimes dangerous because the relationship is forced. The clients can be difficult, uncooperative, negative and often hostile (De Jong and Berg 2001). Therefore, the mandated client has lower levels of motivation for achieving change and hence are less likely to achieve change with more accepting clients. Another problem is that the client may not consider there is a problem to be addressed. For example, a young man mandated to receive social casework services to address offending behavior may deny that they have offended or may justify their actions as a reasonable response because they consider themselves a victim. As a social service work, it is important to consider the different views of the problem can be an obstacle for workers and clients when developing a constructive working relationship.

It does not matter where you are in the world or what type of client you have encountered voluntary, involuntary or mandated, a client is not really a client unless they are willing to participate in the worker/client relationship. A client has to be willing to work with the human service worker in order for this relationship to become established and ultimately maintained. If a client is not receptive to engaging with the worker, this connection will not work. In the many years of working in the human service environment, there is no such thing as a mandated client or an involuntary client, a client has to be open to share their feelings and be compliant to some degree in order for the helping process to work. There has to be a willingness to resolve an issue on the part of the client.

A client is different from a stranger, a friend or a family member who may ask for advice. The advice you may give a family member or friend is free and it is not bounded by any professional standards. It is not bounded by confidentiality; you are not obligated to be non-judgmental or even respectful. The advice given under those circumstances is often tainted with misconceptions, misplaced loyalty and the history of your relationship with this person. Therefore, a client is not a client unless it is under the auspices of a professional relationship and there is an established contract of a working relationship between the worker, the client and the agency.

A Client's Personality

The client is a unique human being with specific nuances such as; their spirit and personality. It is impossible to know the whole person because of the subtle dimensions of a personality and the reorganization between new and old experiences of the personality continuously taking place (Perlman 1957). The client operates as a physical, psychological and social entity that is always processing experiences based on his/her environment (Perlman 1957). The client is ever-changing based on the physical and social environment, past experience, present perceptions and reactions and even future aspirations. The client is also a physical-psychological-social-past-present-future configuration and he/she brings it to every life situation that is encountered (Perlman 1957).

Case Study
Tammy is a 16 year-old Caribbean female of Indian and African descent who is using obscene language, destroying property, attempted homicide of her mother and suicide several times. She is a child of a single parent mother, her father seldom visits. She has been molested by her mother's boyfriends and has been bullied in school. Her personality is based on all these contributing factors.

A human's drive is to gratify basic needs (e.g., Maslow's hierarchy of needs; Maslow1943). The person's behavior directs he/she's specific purpose and meaning whether it is to gain satisfaction, to avoid or dissolve frustration and to maintain a balance in their life (Perlman 1957). The client's behavior affects the ways he/she think, feel and act to achieve that internal sense of comfort or satisfaction which makes him/her feel in tune with the surrounding world and open to a new experience (Perlman 1957). The strength and the particular direction to fulfill one's life's purpose and meaning will differ for different people which, depends on their behavior, energy or culture.

When a traumatic event occurs or an obstacle happens whether it is great or small it will impact clients who will in turn display a range of emotions (e.g., irritation, anxiety or, sadness). Clients make efforts to cope with these new feelings in some way and regain a sense of stability. The coping mechanism is dependent on what the client is willing to do and the mental, physical or social capacity of the client (Perlman 1957). Client's reservoirs of energy have the capacity to think and act in ways calculated to restore a sense of security and relative mastery. Sometimes clients may retreat from difficult situations by relinquishing one goal and pursuing a substitute; sometimes clients may compromise and accommodate the problem or, sometimes clients may attack a problem by strategic maneuvers of thought and action in an effort to solve the problem (Perlman 1957).

The client who comes to an agency for help, he/she has already exhausted other avenues to cope and options to reconcile their feelings. The client arrives and has already reconciled that one of the ways to solve the problem is through little changes in behavior such as the way he/she feels, thinks and acts in the presence of a worker and others. This may be different from his/her behavior outside the casework/client situations. The human service worker may draw inferences as to what the client is striving for and against. By the client's every movement internal and overt, the client is saying "I want something and I act in the ways I can so as to get it, I fear or am blocked by something and I act so as to protect myself against or to manage it" (Perlman 1957). Often the client's behavior reveals that he/she is caught between wanting and fearing, both at once which is the essence of conflict. And sometimes the caseworker will encounter the client who has experienced more frustration than satisfaction in his/her efforts to fulfill life needs and the behavior will show that the client is resigned because they came to the agency. For example, a man who has been experiencing major bouts of depression because of a recent break up with try many alternatives such as; attending religious services, exercising, drinking, using drugs, having sex with multiple partners it is only when the alternatives do not work he may seek an agency for help.

The essence of the casework method is aimed to facilitate the individual's social adaption to restore, reshape or reinforce his/her functioning as a social being (Perlman 1957). The human service worker must understand their purpose is to enable the client to find some effective ways of solving or coping with problems. In order for this to occur, the worker does not necessarily need to take a complete account of each person's dimensions and dynamics but understand the nature of the problem brought for help (e.g., concrete, clinical or, both; Perlman 1957). This will determine what kind of knowledge that is necessary and what aspect of the person needs to be understood.

One of the clearer ways a worker can understand clients is by investigating their personality. Personality is the overall picture of the characteristic behavior of the individual. Behavior includes; thinking, feelings, speaking and doing (Perlman 1957). To know an individual's personality means to inform oneself about the usual way the individual thinks, feels, speaks and does things which are complex is not easily accessible. It requires special knowledge and skills to identify the different aspects of personality growth. The theoretical frameworks of casework method (e.g., Freud Structural Theory, Erikson Psychosocial Stages of Development, and Maslow's Hierarchy of Needs) are some of the more essential theories that can inform a client's personality development. Client's also has beliefs on the belief systems (e.g., ideas, attitudes and expectation about self and others; Schwartz and Lacey 1982). In the Caribbean beliefs in African spiritual practices (e.g., voodoo, obeah) is very present and entrenched in the Caribbean mindset and dictates the client's actions. For example, an elderly lady begins to show signs of dementia and may start exhibiting odd behavior, her daughter may think the lady was possessed by a demon or someone placed voodoo on her and will go to a spiritual healer first before going to see a physician.

Clients also have self-statements which are monologues that influence behavior and feelings (Schwartz and Lacey 1982). In the Caribbean, especially in African household, the responsibility of the family (e.g., the children) is essentially women's business in her roles of a mother, wife and grandmother. It is the self-statement that is substantiated by the culture and is what she tells herself and it will dictate her behavior to care for others before she takes care of herself (Barrow 2000). Finally, all clients have problem-solving and coping mechanisms that have helped the client to survive in the past. In the Caribbean, the roles of the people during slavery or indentureship and colonization have lasted in the family structure of centuries (Barrow 2000). There is an essence of subservience even in female-headed households to a person in a dominant class (e.g., race, gender) the roles and the traditional mechanisms of solving problems are still ingrained in the client, men make the decisions (e.g., uncle, brother) even if it is dangerous for the female. Although the client may have come to the agency for assistance, resorting to the familiar ways of dealing with a problem is hard to resist.

For clients in the Caribbean, it is important to understand the client's personality and interpersonal relationships. All individuals exist in a continually changing world of experience of which they are the center; individuals react to their environment as they experience and perceive it; the client is always striving for stability.

In the Caribbean, historically due to persistent poverty, parents often have to make personal choices to care for children such as giving the children to someone else (e.g., a childless relative or neighbor) to rear while they are seeking income. For the Caribbean client stability in the family both emotionally and financially is very important (Barrow 2000). Behavior is basically a goal-directed attempt of individuals to satisfy their needs as experienced in their mind. Reality for any given individual is the individual's perception of reality. It is important to understand the reality and their perspective of the problem. The best vantage points for understanding behavior is from the client's perspective of themselves because their behavior is usually consistent with the individual's concept of self. Problems arise when a client's concept of self does not match his/her conscious wishes of their behavior and their actual behavior; when there is incongruence between the individual's self-concept and experiences with others it causes a state of anxiety.

Client's Communication Patterns

The Caribbean Perspective of Communication

A client communicates their problem in very different ways and it is important as human service workers to understand the nuances of communication. Human service workers must know how to communicate skillfully with a client in order for the type of relationship to develop in which open client communication can occur. However, clients experience an internal battle of doing the same they have been doing in the past to resolve their issue and resist the worker's assistance although they are coming to the agency. Therefore, human communication is complex and multifaceted. In order for human service workers to help they must understand what the client is communicating. Communication equals information and information can be a new fact which can contrast existing assumptions about the client (Bateson 1979). Information affects how clients and their environment mutually affect each other through feedback. A single unit of communication is a message and an interaction is the exchange of a series of messages between two people (Greene 1996).

Clients have different ways of communicating. There are four axioms of communication (Watzlawick et al. 1967).

- The first is *one cannot communicate*. Even when a client is saying nothing, he or she may be communicating with the worker they are not interested in having a conversation at this time. One can reject, accept or disqualify another's communication just by saying nothing at all. Communication must be clear for there to be a mutual understanding of rejection or acceptance and the Caribbean people are very expressive with non-verbal gestures. Emotions are often conveyed in facial expressions without saying a word.
- When a *client communicates with the worker they are not only conveying a substantive message but they are also making a statement about the definition of the relationship*. A client could be saying I trust you and I will tell you everything or my trust of you is limited and you will find out information on a need to know basis.
- *Communication is qualified by other verbal messages, nonverbal communication of bodily movements, or the context of the communication*. The issue of cause and effect, or blame in relationships is conveyed in the ongoing stream of communication to make sense of their meaning. Each person is truly convinced about the correctness of their own reality and each person in the dialogue is punctuating the sequence of events in their relationship differently. A client may not take personal responsibility for their actions it is important to understand who the client will blame for their own shortcomings.
- *Clients communicate with words and/or posture, gesture, facial expression, voice inflection, the sequence, rhythm, and cadence of words*. These actions can convey progress or if it is a dead end with a client.

Difficulties in relationships arise when communication patterns are in a double-bind situation (Munhall and Bateson 1998) when one person is chronically subjecting the other person to invalidation through a paradoxical interaction. Double –bind dynamics involves one person in power puts down the other person who is a insubordinate in order to maintain power. An intense relationship involving two or more persons with one person in the power position (e.g., parent) and the other person is in the subordinate position (e.g., child) causes anxiety, depression and rage (Bateson et al. 1956). Because it is an intense relationship, it is necessary for the person in the subordinate position to be able to accurately interpret the messages from the person in the power position. Double binding dynamics involve the person in the power position giving the insubordinate position messages, usually verbal about how to feel, think, or behave (e.g., what to do or not do). For example, in order to motivate the child a parent may use punishment or threats of punishment and never rewards, thus creating a learning context based on avoidance or punishment rather than seeking rewards. This sets up a paradigm that the punishment is a withdrawal of love and the client at the same time the parent is giving the child verbal messages the nonverbal messages conflicts with a verbal message. The nonverbal message is communicated by means of posture, gesture, tone of voice, meaningful action and the implications concealed in verbal comments (Bateson et al. 1956). When the client comes to agency part of their despair is the result of a double-bind relationship with people they are familiar with (e.g., family, spouse). In the Caribbean with a rich history of colonization double-bind communication patterns happens daily as people are always vying to exert power over each other. Overall, the clients convey information through their personality and interpersonal relationships and communication patterns. It is important to understand all these dynamics to get to the heart of the problem.

The Problem

Conducting a psychosocial assessment is an assessment of the person's life history, their support systems and presenting problem. One particular student described a client who had a history of child abuse, family abandonment, dropped out of school, unemployment, drug and alcohol abuse. The social work student met the client in a drug rehabilitation program where the client completed his rehabilitation program and was ready to leave the facility. The client was homeless and his girlfriend of 4 years recently left him after he was incarcerated for theft prior to going for rehabilitation. The student asked the client what were his concerns and he said his girlfriend left him because he has a small penis. The client's perception of reality. When I asked the student what was her assessment of the case and what was the presenting problem, the student also said it is because the client has a small penis was the reason for all of his other problems (e.g., child abuse). With all the issues the client had why would that be his presenting problem? What was the student's assessment of the problem to have such a conclusion?

As much as a human service worker can perform miracles; correcting the client's penis size is not one of them. The moral of the story is a problem in a social welfare agency must be something a human service worker can do within your professional responsibility and your agency's purview. At the social agency there are a myriad of problems that are brought to the human service worker's attention such as; addictions, anxiety disorders, autism, child maltreatment, conduct disorders, couple and family problems, depression, developmental disabilities, eating disorders, family violence, gerontology, juvenile delinquency, pain management, phobic disorders, post- traumatic stress, psychosis, sexual deviance, problems of hunger, suicide ideation, or not wanting to die, needing social support or having too much social support. All these and many more come into the social welfare agency. The task of attempting to help with the variety of problems that clients present with is overwhelming.

How a problem is defined largely governs what the worker can do about it (Gitternman 1996). The basic tenet of solving problems is to understand the client and the environment of which the client came from birth to present. Problems clients encounter can be a cause of difficult life transitions, traumatic life events, environmental process, dysfunction, & the transpersonal process.

Life transitions include biological as well as social changes (Gitternman 1996). The physical and biological changes from infancy through puberty and adulthood are universal but the social and cultural expectations associated with the biological condition can cause stress. (disability) People also experience stress from entering new experiences and relationships. It can be physical and biological factors associated with growing older for example. In the Caribbean, people experience stress from entering new experiences and relationships and leaving familiar relationships and environments. Older Caribbean people sometimes migrate to new countries to join their children, acculturation in a new country can cause a lot of stress. Unexpected life transitions (e.g. death) are more stressful than expected ones. Similarly, when life entrances and exits come too early or too late in the life course, they can also be stressful (Gitternman 1996).

Traumatic events due to its suddenness can cause a personal crisis and leave a long-lasting residue of pain. Unexpected death and illness, displacement caused by natural disasters, loss of a cherished home or job are overwhelming and immobilizing. Child sexual abuse in the Caribbean is one of the most under-reported criminal acts against children. Children are often too young to know exactly what is happening to them, but instinctively feel that something is wrong and are often left with the awareness that life will never be the same (Jones 2013). Sexual assault in adults also leaves an indelible mark for both men and women yet it is underreported and never addressed. The long term effects of sexual abuse in girls have been researched and understood to leave psychological conflicts for the victims which leads to problems bought to the agency (e.g., prostitution, drug abuse; Jones 2013).

Environmental pressures can also cause problems for clients. The social and physical environment provides essential instrumental resources and emotional support to the tasks of daily living (Valentich and Gripton 1994). They can also create significant troubles and distress. In Haiti, the 2010 earthquake caused irreparable damage with over 100,000 deaths and millions of dollars of damaged infrastructure (USAID 2010). This has caused quite a bit of psychological distressed to the people who are left behind to survive. The problem may be some unmet-economic, medical, educational, recreational which hampers or undermines a person quality of life. Or it may be one of stress-psychological, social, physical which causes the person to be ineffective or disturbed in carrying out his social roles (Gitternman 1996).

Dysfunctional interpersonal processes are concerned with problematic internal family or group relationships and communication patterns that exacerbate existing stress and /or become yet another painful stressor in people's lives. Dysfunctional family and group processes are expressed in double-bind communication (e.g., one with power speaking derogatively down to the one with less power) and behaviors such as scapegoating and hostility (Valentich and Gripton 1994).

With this knowledge of the type of problem the client is experiencing, the worker is able to understand all the dimensions of the problem and the client can begin to rectify the problem (Perlman 1957). The problems under the purview of social casework are those which vitally affect or are affected by a person's social functioning. Whether such needs and stress occur singularly or in combination it is the person's inability to muster the means by which to maintain or achieve social comfort and adequacy which brings the problem within the locus of the casework's concern (Perlman 1957).

This focus upon the problems a client is encountering in his/her social secureness and functional adequacy is one distinguishing mark of social casework (Gitternman 1996; Perlman 1957). It implies that the primary focus of the social caseworker's help is upon the difficulties the person is having in behaving in socially accepted or constructive ways or upon the assaults he/she is experiencing from the circumstances. The client of the worker typically sees his/her problems as lying in some interacting relationship between the client and some other person or between the client and his/her circumstances. The help the client seeks typically for some readjustment of the self, or in relation to the demands and expectations of the social role he/she carries as a spouse, parent, and student. The client wants help in the readjustment of some parts of his/her social situation so he/she can maintain or achieve the equilibrium necessary for daily pursuits. Reference

Overall, the problem is the focus of the casework method, the goal is to resolve the problems and not necessarily change the person. However, sometimes in order to resolve the problem the person has to change their behavior, beliefs and personality. But there have to be special qualities of the worker in order for this process to begin.

The Worker

The exceptional social service workers are able to convey genuineness and kindness in every interaction with a client. The values of a social service worker working with clients should include (Boy and Pine 1983):

- Valuing the worth of a person;
- responsible action occurs within the context of respect for the dignity and worth of others;
- you must have a fundamental respect for the client's freedom to know, shape, and determine personal attitudes and behavior;
- the client possesses free will, and is the determiner of personal destiny;
- a person's free functioning not only tends toward the development of the self but also includes a responsibility to other persons;
- the client enhances the self by fulfilling obligations to his/herself and others;
- the client begins to relate to others with a sense of personal responsibility and ethical behavior;
- love and peace are basic strivings and must be advanced during one's lifetime.

There are some basic behaviors and characteristics that make a human service worker more appealing than others. Similarly, in the worker-client situation, certain behavior and personal qualities that human service workers tend to nurture in interpersonal relationships can put clients at ease and make them feel important and cared about.

Providing Warmth

A human service worker should convey warmth which involves a feeling of interest, concern, well-being, and affection toward the client as a feeling in human interaction. Conveying warmth also involves enhancing the positive feelings of one person toward another. Warmth demonstrates acceptance when it is shown to be respectful of the client with valuing statements (e.g., 'you must be upset') and enthusiasm with the client's rendition of the story (e.g., looking like you are interested in the story). Warmth can be communicated to the client both verbally and nonverbally specifically with facial expressions.

Facial Expressions

Facial expressions provide an excellent movement of communication (Kirst-Ashman and Hull 2014). Facial expressions are executed with facial muscles. Facial expressions can be used to reinforce what is said verbally and corroborate the fact that you mean what you say. It is important that as human service workers; you are aware of your facial responses so that you know what you are communicating and make certain that your facial expressions correspond with both your other types of nonverbal behavior (e.g. hand gestures) and with what you are saying verbally. Giving a client a mixed message by saying one thing while looking like you mean another is not helpful, such action can convey doubt that you are being truthful.

Empathy and Genuineness

Empathy enhances the worker-client relationship and it is essential to the helping process. Empathy involves not only being in tune with how a client feels but also conveying to that client that you understand how he/she feels without words. It does not necessarily mean you think the client's feelings are positive or negative, nor does it mean that you are having the same feelings yourself. Empathy is purely an acknowledgment that you understand the client's situation. Clients who feel you have listened to how they feel and they are you not against them are much more likely to be willing to work with you toward finding solutions to problems. Empathy communicates to the client that you are there to help solve the problem. Empathizing with positive emotions can also be helpful. Empathic responding may elicit feelings and discussion about previously unmentioned issues. Empathy provides the worker with a means of getting at feelings that are not expressed verbally. Empathy also makes making confrontations less hostile.

Genuineness is the honest, natural and open expression of yourself. Genuineness simply means that you continue to be yourself despite the fact that you are working to accomplish goals as a social service worker. Personality refers to the unique configuration of qualities and attributes that make you an individual but clients often tell me that I am genuine because I am real and forthright in my opinion and approach.

In the Caribbean to be genuine, is it important to be yourself and convey empathy without being condescending towards the client. It is important to show similarities with the client's life story and to let them understand they are not alone in the journey they are walking but others have walked this journey too.

Body Movements

Body movement and positioning can provide information to the client that you are either too rigid or intense. Body tension involves how rigid or tense muscles appear when you position yourself and more frequently coincides with emotional tension. Such tension can be demonstrated by sitting perfectly straight and allowing minimal movement of extremities. Tension is also apparent when a person makes quick nervous gestures such as continuously tapping your foot. The opposite of a tense stance is a relaxed one. Relaxation can be portrayed by slow, loose movements and a decidedly casual, informal presentation of self. The more extreme form of a relaxed stance would probably to lie down. Ideally presenting somewhere in between the two extremes is best. To some extent, body positioning is a matter of personal style. You need to appear genuine that is they you are reflecting aspects of your true individual personality. The nonverbal behavior of body positioning by facial expressions, hand movements, eye contact, the manner in which you sit, and how close you stand next to a client matters in the helping process and providing personal space.

Active Listening

Attentive listening is not that simple. First, the distinction must be made between hearing and listening. Listening implies more than just audio reception of words that are said. It focuses on comprehending the meaning of what is said. Third, there may be environmental barriers impeding communication of the message. Listening is an essential characteristic that is once active, attentive and purposeful. The purpose of listening is to understand the client words and feelings as accurately as possible. It is important to have the mental concentration to pay attention to what is said and what is not said and what is suggested. As a human service worker, listening is a conscious activity that helps in the practice of accepting the client and the information they are providing. Aspects of effective listening is to maintain eye contact with the client during conversations (Kirst-Ashman and Hull 2014). The human service worker's eye contact with the client helps to direct the clients physical and mental attention towards the client. When interacting with the client, the worker's mind should be clear of preconceived ideas and opinion of the client. Anxieties or apprehension about the interview must be brought to the level of awareness and should be resolved. If they cannot be resolved immediately, they should be consciously kept aside for the time being. The worker's ear should be trained to listen to everything that the client says. What the client says or what he/she appears to be cannot but evoke thinking in the mind of the worker, but thinking in this context should not deflect or sidetrack from the client. In other words, the worker should be capable of disciplined thinking that helps him/her to understand what the client says to make a mental note of what the client does not say and to ask appropriate questions.

Obstacles to listening are distraction of various kinds that take a listener off the path of active listening. There can be external distractions in the form of noises in the environmental and other people talking. Internal distractions are one owns thoughts, connected or unconnected with the worker or the subject matter the client's speech. Sometimes the speaker's statements may bring to the listener's remembrance similar experiences and set the mind off, away from the path of listening. The listener's anxiety or fear concerning the speaker can become a block to good listening. When the worker is anxious that his/her response to the speaker should be appropriate his/her mind gets pre-occupied with the formulation of the response. This obstacle occurs frequently in the worker-client contact, where the worker is anxious that should be able to win the clients confidence and that he should use the correct words in front of the client. A worker who is anxious about empathizing with the client may be turning over in his/her mind the different words and ways of showing empathy while the client is speaking. So instead of focusing attention on how he should respond when this happens the workers' response may not necessarily suit the context. Through statements like "I understand your feelings", 'It is natural to have such feelings.' Selective listening which refers to the mental tendency of hearing only what one like to hear, prevents effective listening. In ordinary conversation, a considerable amount of information gets turned out of hearing because of selective listening. A client may tune out of a conversation conscious or not so consciously when emotionally painful or unpleasant things are being spoken even by the client or the worker. The client may say something vague. The sender's intent may not be the same as the impact on the receiver. In summary, listening is not easy. It demands concentration, perceptiveness, and the use of a range of interviewing skills.

Building Trust

One of the important features as a human service worker must accomplish is building trust. Trust is earned by the human service worker from the client it is what makes your warmth, genuineness, and empathy believable. There are four components to trust; integrity, intent, capabilities and results (Convey 2006). Integrity is being congruent inside and out meant and that you mean what you say and saying what you mean. Integrity is the courage to act in accordance with your values and beliefs. The second core to trust is intent. Trust grows when our motives are straightforward and based on mutual benefit. There is no hidden agenda or someone we don't believe they are acting in our best interest. We are suspicious about everything that says or do. The third core of trust is capabilities. There are abilities we have that inspire confidence in our talents, attitudes, skills, knowledge, and style. They are the means we use to produce results. The fourth core for trust is results. This refers to our track record our performance, our getting the right things done. If we don't accomplish what we are expected to do, it diminishes one's credibility.

For example, in Jamaica, Jamaicans have a healthy distrust of those in authority and prefer to put their faith in those they know well, such as their extended family and close friends who are treated as if they were family. This can be seen in the fact that many still prefer to form a form of informal banking instead of securing a loan called a "partner" (it is also done in other Caribbean islands called other terms such as, 'su su'). A partner is a financial arrangement between friends and neighbors. Each person in the group agrees to contribute a set amount into the partner for a specific number of weeks. Accumulated funds are used to make down payments for large purchases such as buying a house or a business. The basic requirement of the partner is trust. To become a member of the elite group, a person must be recommended by a friend or relative. These components of trust are the line between the client, the worker, the agency and success in helping.

Empowerment

In the Caribbean, where the majority of the population is people of color (e.g., African, Asian, Indian, Latino) a tool social service workers should know and utilize is the empowerment approach. The empowerment approach provides a historical perspective of a client's ethnic/psychosocial cultural history of oppression and the structural perspective which relates to how does your background are barriers to progression. Understanding the historical background of your client enables the working people of color, women, and those who are oppressed by virtue of sexual orientation, physical and mental challenges youth or age and help them confront the obstacles imposed by class, race, and differences. The empowerment approach makes the connection between the client and social and economic justice.

The worker in the empowerment approach is a real person who has awareness of her or his own experiences of oppression and/or membership in the oppressor group. This awareness begins with the client's self-awareness and goes beyond this to having a raised consciousness about oppression itself and an ability to share this in the helping proves through self-disclosure. There is no mysticism about the helper or the helping process. The stance is 'side by side' and an authentic presentation of self. The helping process itself is shared with the client initially and as the process unfolds.

The Agency

Social service agencies or human service agencies are where clients typically come for help with his/her problems. It is the largest employer for human service workers which are in schools, hospitals, government agencies, courts, child protection agencies, to name a few. All of these agencies have been established to achieve certain broad purposes such as provide services or goods, where human service workers play an integral part in its operation. Its purpose is to help clients with a range of social problems and alleviate barriers that hamper the client's quality of life. The type of social service agencies differ but fall within one of three categories: their source of financial support which can include the government or private funding; the agencies' full authority to disseminate services is under the auspices of the agency (e.g., arms of government like ministry) or a secondary agency which derives their authority and responsibility from the host agency (e.g., a non-profit agency of the United Nations such as UNICEF); last the agencies' mission is related to how they provide services for example if it is in the court system, the social services provided will be legal related matters.

Perlman (1957) outlined in her seminal book *The Casework Process*, characteristics of an agency (e.g., food, shelter, health). An agency embodies a society's decision to protect its members against social breakdowns, to prevent their maladjustments and to promote the development of better human functioning. The agency is developed to deal with a social problem by addressing particular areas of need. The agency's mission and vision detail its function to provide help. The structure of an agency identifies and assigns separate and joint responsibilities, authorities and tasks to each person and demarcates the relationship among various functions in the agency. The ways and means which an agency effectively provides help depends on financial resources, the consistency between ascertained needs and proffered means, the knowledge and competency of the agency's staff and the support of the community.

An agency has two kinds of expectations: the professional and the bureaucratic. Large social service agencies have large internal organizational systems and bureaucratic expectations which includes; acceptance of authority, specialization of tasks and efficient mechanisms to carry out tasks. In agencies with a bureaucracy, there is a hierarchy of decision-making power and collegial relationships with an emphasis on meeting client's need and allowing for client self-determination and individualization. Professional expectations call for commitment to professional values and to the service of clients. Before a worker can effectively deliver service as a professional in a bureaucratic organization, the worker must first understand the organization and define the agency's boundaries (e.g., work within the scope of the agencies guidelines) and determine the environmental factors that influence the structure and functioning of the agency. Overall, human service workers not only need to understand the agency in which they are employed but they also need to be able to understand other social agencies in order to help the clients utilize the resources and services of other agencies (Perlman 1957).

The social service agency's organizational structure is made up of many members with different purposes and powers, all dependent upon one another in the organization. Every staff member's professional commitment and skill in an agency works to carry out the agency's mission and function. The worker must identify with the purpose and policies of the agency. The human service worker represents the agency in its individualized problem-solving help process and practices with a conviction that the client's welfare is the purpose. The worker in the agency maintains a social conscience and conducts his/herself ethically and professionally.

The social service agency is a living, adaptable organism susceptible to being understood and changed, much as other living organisms. The most important aspect of agency function is that it constitutes the meeting point of the worker and the client and it is the place that brings them together and gives meaning and sustenance to their continued contact. The agency must be adaptable to the changing social problems in a country. It must embrace immigrants and displaced persons if this issue becomes a relevant problem. The agency is often an office or building and is the immediate environment of the worker-client interaction. Even when a human service worker makes home visits or meets with the client in other environments the influence (e.g., rules or regulations) of the agency is prominent and the interaction between the client and worker must be under the purview and guidelines of the agency.

The community provides finances and sanctions for the agency to exist. Community attitudes impact the agency and its capacity to deliver services. If the community does not want an orphanage to exist in the community it can make it very difficult to operate in that community and obtain police support for example.

In the nations with smaller populations such as the Caribbean, throughout the region there are a low proportion of trained social workers among the service providers (Maxwell 1994). Many human service worker's functions are performed by untrained personnel but there are also some undertaken by persons with other qualifications which are given some measure of recognition (e.g., management, accountancy). Rehabilitative services are offered in the areas of Family and Child Welfare, Corrections, Substance Abuse and in the field of Mental Health (Maxwell 1994). Some primary agencies are government funded (e.g., hospitals, welfare offices) but a number of small nongovernmental organizations (NGO), also offer services (e.g. domestic violence agencies), especially for children and families. The shortcomings of most of the rehabilitation and developmental services are as follows: they are usually inadequately staffed and insufficient to serve the client's demand and the need for service. Documentation in certain services is decidedly limited and, in most, little or no attention is given to research. With very few exceptions, effective advocacy to impact policy-making is absent.

Regional governments in the Caribbean all offer programs of youth development and leadership training to promote community development/community economic development projects but they are rare outcomes oriented to see if these programs are truly beneficial. There is also a very low proportion of trained social workers offering services in most agencies and salaries are almost uniformly poor. The rate of trained personnel is high, with persons either moving to human resource management roles in the industrial sector or joining other poorly paid professionals by immigrating to developed countries (Maxwell 1994).

Review Questions

1. What is important to know when working with mandated clients?
2. Why is it important to understand the client's personality?
3. What is so important about the presenting problem?
4. Why is your facial expression important in the casework method?
5. How important is active listening to the therapeutic relationship?
6. Why is empowerment so important in the casework method?

References

Barrow, C. (2000). *Family in the Caribbean*. Jamaica: Ian Randle Publishers.

Bateson, G. (1979). *Mind and nature: A necessary unity*. New York: E.P. Dutton.

Bateson, G., Jackosn, D., Haley, J., & Weakland, J. (1956). Toward a theory of schizophrenia. *Behavioral Science, 1*, 251–264.

Boy, A., & Pine, G. (1983). Counseling: Fundamentals of theoretical renewal. *Counseling and Values, 27*, 248–255. https://doi.org/10.1002/j.2161-007X.1983.tb01140.

Convey, S. (2006). *The speed of trust*. New York: Free press, ltd.

De Jong, P., & Berg, I. (2001). Co-constructing cooperation with mandated clients. *Social Work, 46*(4), 361–374.

Gitternman, A. (1996). Ecological perspective, response to professor Jerry Wakefield. *Social Service Review, 70*(2), 472–475.

Greene, G. J. (1996). An integrative dialectical-pragmatic approach to time-limited treatment: Working with unemployed clients as a case in point. In A. R. Roberts (Ed.), *Managing crisis and brief treatment* (pp. 160–194). Chicago: Nelson-Hall.

Jones, A. (2013). *Understanding child sexual abuse: Perspectives from the Caribbean*. London: Palgrave Macmillan.

Kirst-Ashman, K., & Hull, G. (2014). *Understanding generalist practice* (7th ed.). Australia: Cernage Learning/Palgrave Macmillan.

Maslow, A. H. (1943). A theory of human motivation. *Psychological Review, 50*(4), 370–396. https://doi.org/10.1037/h0054346. *via* psychclassics.yorku.ca.

Maxwell, J. A. (1994, October). Social work and social issues: The caribbean. In *Center for International Social Work: Inaugural Conference* (p. 4).

Munhall & Bateson (1998). The moving face during speech communication. In Campbell, R.; Dodd. B.; Burnham, d. (Ed.), *Hearing by Eye II* (pp. 123–142). United Kingdom: Psychology Press.

Perlman, H. H. (1957). *Social casework: A problem solving process*. Chicago: The University of Chicago Press.

Schwartz, B., & Lacey, L. (1982). *Behaviorism, science and human nature*. New York: Norton Books.

USAID. (2010). Haiti earthquake: Crisis and response. Congressional Research Service.

Valentich, M. & Gripton, J. (1994). Making decisions about dual relationships. Paper presented at the Conference on Sexual Exploitation by Health Professionals and Clergy. Toronto.

Watzlawick, P., Beavin, J., & Jackson, D. (1967). *Pragmatics of human communication: A study of interactional pattersn, pathologies and paradoxes*. New Yok: W.W. Norton.

Chapter 7
The Helping Process

Highlights of this Chapter:

- The importance of the interview.
- How to prepare an interview using the casework method.
- An overview of Verbal and non-verbal communication.
- steps of data collection in the casework method

The Interview

A place to start when learning how to interview and work with individual clients is to examine the skills of how to establish a good worker-client relationship. Although the client is a stranger to the agency and this may be the first visit to the agency, the worker has to build a rapport with the client quickly to gather data regarding the problem and how the client perceives it, what has been done about the problem, gather some data about the client, their family and resources/support systems. As a worker you are there to help your client clearly identify what the problems are and what can be done to solve it. The skilful way the worker conducts the interview may be of help to the client in terms of the concern, hope, warmth and interest conveyed to the client, which in turn starts a process, sooner or later, within the client to mobilize inner resources of the client for problem-solving.

Part of the social casework method is the helping interview. An important component to helping is the utility of communicating accurate empathy, authenticity and positive regard in the helping process is conveyed through components of the helping interview which will help skills development and should be acceptable to workers, they need to be expanded and adapted to fit a wide variety of casework situations and circumstances.

In the casework method, the meeting between the worker and the client in a face-to-face conversation is essential to begin the client-worker relationship with

E. J. Johnson, C. L. Huggins, *Social Casework Methodology: A Skills Handbook for the Caribbean Human Services Worker*, SpringerBriefs in Social Work,
https://doi.org/10.1007/978-3-030-27319-4_7

client (Kirst-Ashman and Hull 2014). Interviews are about the communication of the client's problems, solutions to the problem encourage positive change and promote client well-being (Kirst-Ashman and Hull 2014). It is not a casual conversation but a professional activity on the part of the human service worker because the conversation is geared for a specific purpose which is to obtain information from the client and assess the client's problem and related issues or situations as well as, give help (Kirst-Ashman and Hull 2014). The emphasis of the interview is to plan action. As a worker, you are there to help the client clearly identify what the problems are and what can be done to solve them.

Interviewing is a two-way process in which the worker is receiving knowledge from the client (e.g., the problem and history of the client) and imparting information to the client (e.g., official procedures of the agency and the role of the worker; Kirst-Ashman and Hull 2014). The information the worker gathers from the client is sorted and analyzed between what is relevant aspects linked to form a verbal picture of the problem and provides the indications of cause- effect. During this process the worker applies the knowledge of social sciences for understanding the behavior of the client and their support systems (e.g., family, friends) who may have accompanied the client to the agency (Kirst-Ashman and Hull 2014).

Communication with a client is a core skill for interviewing. An interview is a conversation with a deliberate purpose that the client is willing to participate in it resembles a conversation in many ways that both involve verbal and nonverbal communication (Kirst-Ashman and Hull 2014). Interviews are more than just a pleasant conversation because they have a specified purpose. This purpose is to exchange information systematically with a view toward illuminating and solving problems, promoting growth or planning strategies or actions aimed at improving the quality of life for people. An interview is also a formal structure where the role of the participants are clear; time is predetermined by client and worker; and location is understood. The formal structure and role involved are based on the role of the worker as a professional and serious helper. The client assumes the role of one needing assistance and assuming the unilateral focus of attention, concern, and help. The interview's formal structure involves time constraints, appointment times and location (e.g., agency, home visit). The interview's process in terms of what transpires is to engage with the client, assess the problem and situation and create an intervention with the client involved (Kirst-Ashman and Hull 2014).

During the interview the worker has to convey warmth, empathy and genuineness to help foster professional relationships with clients. The emphasis is on planning and action. As a worker, you are there to help your client clearly identify what the problems are and what can be done to solve them.

Interview Preparation

Specific suggestions for starting and subsequently conducting the interview happens before the interview and to prepare for the interview the worker needs to think ahead about four important variables. First is there pertinent demographic information that will be needed such as addresses, phone numbers, next of kin, age, gender information. This will help you to contact the client for future meetings. This will help you to contact the client for future interviews. Second, anticipate any questions the client might ask that you (the worker) should be prepared for (e.g., what is your role in the agency). The interview's period should be clearly specified such as, when the interview is scheduled to begin and when it needs to end. The meeting should start punctually (Kirst-Ashman and Hull 2014). Making the client wait beyond the scheduled starting time may imply that the client's time is not important and that you have better things to do. A timely start conveys common courtesy and respect for the client. The interview should have timely ending and the next client should not be kept waiting. When the worker wants to end the interview alert the client by reminding them of the time and when the interview is supposed to end. The fourth variable that needs consideration prior to the interview is the interview's purpose. Preparation involves specifying the interview's purpose and translating goals into specific items that needed to be covered.

Initial introductions during the interview are a combination of formal and informal interactions. Names are exchanged with typical pleasantries such as 'it nice to meet you' or any warm greeting. Using surnames of the client is usually best since they imply greater respect. Handshakes are also often appropriate. However, you need to be aware of the client's level of comfort and anxiety. If a client cringes as you extend your hand, nonchalantly take it back and continue with a verbal interchange. When beginning the interview, initiating brief innocuous exchanges about some bland topic such as the weather or a current event may also be appropriate. A short interchange can be used to soften the formal edge of the interview and make the situation warmer.

During the interview it is important to think about how the client must feel coming into the initial interview with the worker. The client maybe nervous and wondering will the worker interrogate or criticize the client's decisions. Many clients will approach the interview with anxiety others however may arrive with resentment or hostility it is important to know the difference. The important thing is for you to pay close attention to their verbal and nonverbal behavior.

Verbal and Non-Verbal Communication

Human interaction and communication involve both verbal and nonverbal behavior. Verbal behavior is what is being said, non-verbal behavior is communication in ways other than spoken words. People communicate by facial expressions, hand movements, eye contact, the manner in which they sit and how close they stand to you. Any aspect of a person's presence that conveys ideas or information without being spoken is non-verbal communication. Eye contact is important when establishing rapport with clients. However, the appropriate type and amount of eye contact vary depending upon the client's cultural background. Holding your head straight and facing clients during interviews conveys to them that they are important and then you are listening to what they are saying.

In the Caribbean, for example in Jamaica (Commiscei 2017) it is important to recognize these verbal and non-verbal cues in preparation and during an interview: Jamaicans (like most Caribbean islands) are outwardly warm and friendly, the people often appear standoffish at the initial introduction because they are reserved until they get to know someone, the most common greeting is the handshake with direct eye contact, and a warm smile and using the appropriate salutation for the time of day: "good morning", "good afternoon", or "good evening"; it is imperative to show deference and respect to those in positions of authority, address people by their honorific title (Mr., Mrs., or Miss) and their surname until a personal relationship has developed; status is respected in Jamaica. It is quite common to hear someone referred to as " bossman" or "bosswoman" when the person is addressing them is an employee; appointments are necessary and easy to schedule meetings and will have a friendly tone even though they can be somewhat formal, expect some small talk before business is discussed and let the Caribbean client decide when it is time to speak about the issue, Caribbean client expect punctuality although they are not always successful at arriving on time themselves. Once a relationship has been established, women may hug and kiss on each cheek, starting with the right and men often pat each other's shoulder or arm during the greeting process or while conversing. Caribbean clients can be direct communicators and are not afraid to say what they think, even if they disagree with what you have said. They value logic and linear thinking at the same time they value tact and sensitivity and dislike overt aggression. These pointers and continuous contact with the client will lead to relationship building.

Place of Interview

Interviews may occur in a variety of settings, depending on the type of agency. Some interviews take place in hospitals or schools. Many occur in the worker's office, which gives the worker control over the positioning of the desk and chairs to enhance the client's comfort level. Workers need to be sensitive to the overall impression of the office environment itself. Putting personal pictures and trinkets may not be appropriate for a professional environment (Kirst-Ashman and Hull 2014).

Some interviews may take place in the client's home which provides the advantage of seeking where and how he or she lives. However, home visits may have a disadvantage for the client because of the distractions in the home (e.g., children, pets, television). Home visits should be at a time that is convenient for the client. Often a convenient time may not be during the day, evening, or even weekends. In such cases having a job that is flexible in scheduling your work time is helpful.

Home visits can be scheduled by phone. During the initial conversation, you should identify who you are, clearly state the purpose of the visit. Some clients will not have phones, which makes arranging for a visit more difficult. You might ask the client to notify you for the best available time to meet (Kirst-Ashman and Hull 2014). Considering your safety when visiting various communities is important.

As a worker you must weigh the extent to which you need or are required to make a home visit against the potential danger in which it will place you in.

Doing a risk assessment should be a part of your thinking when you are working away from your office. This might include environmental factors (e.g., lack of transportation) that could threaten you from getting to and from your appointment as well as potential threats from other people. This could include clients with a history of violence, stalkers, people currently using drugs or alcohol or those who experience mental illnesses. Knowing something about one's client ahead of time is one way of assessing the risk involved. During a home visit if a volatile situation arises these are a few suggestions (Kirst-Ashman and Hull 2014):

- *Remain outwardly calm regardless of how you feel inside.*
- *Do not show anger, anxiety.*
- *Remain respectful toward the individual who is threatening*
- *Continue to face the aggressor do not turn your back away from them.*
- *Use a calm voice in talking with the individual.*
- *If the client is standing ask time to sit down to talk with you.*
- *Avoid defensiveness or taking the person's anger personally.*
- *Be honest in what you say and do not try to promise something you cannot deliver.*
- *Use appropriate empathy toward the individual's feelings.*
- *If de-escalation is not working, remove yourself from the situation.*

Observation

Observation is the practice of noticing features about people, things or situations, and in the context of casework, the purpose is to use the observed data for an understanding of the client and their situation. The worker has to take cognizance of the following with reference to the client (Kirst-Ashman and Hull 2014):

1. The general outward appearance.
2. The facial expression, posture, gesture.
3. The characteristics, particularly the emotional nuances of interactions that take place between clients and others, including their family members.

The worker should not have any difficulty in paying attention to the client's personal appearance his/her clothes, level of cleanliness. Generally, the clothes are indicative of the client's socio-economic class, but there are expectations. There have been instances where the relatives of patients have appeared in shabby clothes with the intention of hiding their socio-economic status in contexts where certain payments or to qualify for welfare benefits. There is also cases of clients who are more concerned about their clothes than about giving nutritious food to their children. Some of the poorest clients present a neat and tidy in appearance through their clothes may be almost threadbare with repeated washing.

The human face occasionally reflects the feelings within and to the worker facial expression is a matter for observation. Feelings like sadness, anger and hostility do not need verbal expression to indicate their presence there will be tell-tale signs on the face that bespeak the unexpressed feelings. Similarly, the individual's postures, gestures, tone of voice and body movements are also meaningful.

The client who sits on the edge of their chair may be doing so because of their feelings of strangeness or nervousness. Many clients do not feel comfortable on their first day of visit to an agency. The pressure of their problems that they are having to talk to a stranger about it add to their discomfiture. The confusion and tension that the client experiences within is likely to make him fidgety and restless. The way the client sits and the manner in which the client participates in the conversation with the worker should be observed carefully for indications of the client's emotional state of mind whether the client is tense or relaxed, trusting on suspicious, receptive or inattentive. Knowing what the client feels or getting at least some clues to the client's feelings is helpful in that the worker can prime him/herself to respond appropriately. For instance, a client who feels ill at ease can be helped to feel more comfortable.

The clients themselves may be putting on a façade to test the worker's attitude. It is not a rare experience for workers working with adolescents of correctional institutions to see nothing but boredom and indifference in the demeanour of the young clients with whom they are trying to hold a conversation. It may turn out that the client's indifference is put on, in an attempt to test out the worker's authenticity, insofar as the client's declaration of interest in the client is concerned.

Mannerism and habitual body movements are also significant. When there is an open expression of emotions like shedding tears, the pathos behind the action is understandable. However, when a person weeps repeatedly over the same event, or situation there is a possibility that the individual besides expressing sadness, is also using the occasion for an additional purpose, though not on a conscious level.

The body mind relationship is manifest in the body movements which give expressions of feelings. This phenomenon is appropriately called body language and may or may out be accompanied by verbal expression. What happens in the case of body language is that it is non-verbal communication, but it is involuntary communication or transmission of messages, without any volition on the part of the communicator. The message of information mostly about feelings. The speaker may want to conceal information about the feelings that he experiences, nevertheless the information leaks through. For instance, tears may gush out depending on the intensity of the feelings, regardless of the fact that the person does not want to be seen weeping. Likewise, the emotional material that seeps out of the mind on the face of the individual is clearly visible to others, though invisible to the client. Since gestures and facial expressions are involuntary in real life situations in a play the actors enacting a role on the stage does not experience in real life the feelings of the person who is being portrayed in that role, but the client imagine the feelings and consequently project the client as having those feelings. On occasions when congruence is lacking between verbal and non-verbal communications, it may be surmised that the person is deliberately hiding behind words. Take for instance the context in which a man is talking about the business failure of another man who has been his rival in business. The speaker is expressing verbally his sympathy for the man and his sadness that such adversity has befallen him. What appears on the speakers' face is however a mischevious smile and some signs of gratification. The discrepancy between his verbal assertion and non-verbal communication is due to the fact that he does not want to reveal the feelings of gratification that his experiences within, since the feelings are quite strong signs of them appear on the client's face.

Worker-Client Relationship

The worker-client relationship is another casework tool that needs to be delineated. Relationship between any two people is the condition of their being connected in a significant way. As stated earlier the worker-client relationship is a professional relationship that it has to be positive in nature. Only a positive relationship can serve as a means towards the desirable end for the client. Professional relationships are bound by time and specific purposes. When the purpose is met, the relationship comes to an end. The worker-client relationship has some special characteristics. Though it is attached to a specific purpose or purposes it entails dealing with the tangible and concrete areas of living as well as the intangible area of emotions.

Communication in the interview is the process of transmitting information and messages between two people or more. The worker-client relationship is interdependent in the sense that communication skills on the part of the worker initiate a positive relationship and a positive relationship facilitates constructive communication between the worker and the client. The evolvement of the relationship depends on two persons, it is incumbent on the worker to use his/her expertise to initiate a positive relationship with the client. Granting that the worker makes the correct approach it does not always follow that the client responds positively. There are people who for some reason or other are unable to relate to people. Perhaps their life experiences (e.g., child sexual abuse) are such that they are unable to trust other people. There are some who have been repeatedly let down by the important people of their lives. There are others whose meaningful relationships could be cut short through death or other circumstances. Clients whose personality has been marred by unhappy events related to their personal relationships may be unable to respond to the worker's overtures of friendship.

Building Rapport

Rapport is an important phenomenon in social casework. The word rapport is used to refer to the positive nature of the worker-client relationship. The worker may look for the following signs of rapport with reference to his/her relationship with the client (Kirst-Ashman and Hull 2014).

1. The client shows interest in meeting the worker and keeps appointments.
2. The client expresses his/her feelings during the course of interviews.
3. The client participates adequately in the interviews, talking about his/her, experiences and relationships.
4. The client indicates a degree of commitment to action.

The depth of the worker-client relationship varied from case to case. In many cases this is built on the rapport. While interviewing the worker is listening, observing and communicating. The connection between the relationship and communication has already been pointed out. To put it in a nutshell, casework tools are interlinked dynamically to produce certain desirable outcomes.

Data Collection Methods

One important aspect of the casework method is data collection because you need to have enough information to make a comprehensive and qualified decision. In the casework method data or client information and how it is gathered and analyzed depends on many factors, including the context, the issue that needs to be monitored, the purpose of the data collection and the nature of the problem. In the interest of effectiveness and efficiency, it is recommended that efforts be made to collect data that will shed light on issues or opportunities. To protect the credibility and reliability of data, information should be gathered using accepted data collection techniques. The following are steps of data collection in the casework method:

The first step is to identify the presenting problems, issues and/or opportunities for collecting data and to decide what next steps to take. To do this, it may be helpful to conduct a personal assessment of the client and any other information needed from persons in the environment (Johnson 2017). The social service worker must decide when and how to collect information to achieve certain goals. They must create non-exhaustive questions to collect as much information possible. Part of the data collection is an interview that covers the person's life for the duration of existence of an individual. A lifespan data collection allows the social service worker to analyze the client through the theoretical lens of Freud's (1926) structural theory, psychosocial influences and the human life cycle (Erikson 1950), social and environmental determinant of behavior (e.g., Maslow's Hierarchy of Needs, Ecosystem, Family systems). A life span data collection tool is most appropriate to get information about the client's birth, childhood experiences, developmental milestones, family circumstances, education obtainment, occupational experience and relationships throughout the life. The exhaustive questions that are needed to obtain information about a client's life history should cover events that occur during the client's timeline, developmental milestones, the quality of relationships among family members and any other events that are of importance to the problem that the client may present. Below is an example of the lifespan interview format.

Lifespan Interview

Childhood

1. What is your date of birth?
2. What is your gender?
3. What is your ethnicity?
4. Name your parents, are they alive or deceased.
   a. Did you live and grow up with your parents? If not with who did you grow up with?
   b. Were they married, what was their relationship like?
   c. Were they good parents.
   d. Did you trust your mother?
   e. Did you trust your father?
5. If you requested something from your parents, what were your expectations?
6. How many siblings do you have?
   a. What are their names?
   b. What are their age?
   c. What are their genders
   d. Did you trust and support your siblings, which were you closest too and which ones you were not close to and why not?.
7. Growing up what was the structure of your home (e.g., wooden, concrete)
8. Growing up what was your neighborhood like?
9. Growing up what was your religion. Did you attend religious services? How often.
10. What school did you go to in primary school?
11. Did you enjoy school? Did you get good grades, if not why not?
12. Did anything significant happen from birth to 11 years old?

Adolescence

13. Did you have any friends, did you have any problems making friends?
14. Did anything significant happen during your adolescence with your parents, siblings, other family members, friends?
15. Did you have a romantic relationship with anyone, how did you meet?
16. Did you like school, did you get good grades, if you did not why?
17. Did you do sport or any other activities?
18. Did you have any friends, did you have any problems making friends?
19. Did you have any passes to pass for university or some other school?
20. What did you want to be when you grew up?
21. If you requested something from your parents, what were your expectations?

22. How was your community? Were you in a gang? Did you start doing drugs or alcohol? What age did this occur?
23. When you were an adolescent, did you remember assessing your strengths and weaknesses? What were your strengths or weaknesses?
24. Did you have a lot of peer group involvement?
25. In adolescence, what were your goals for adulthood?
26. When you were an adolescent, what was so important in your life that you are willing to commit to it?

Young Adulthood (Ages 19–30)

27. Did you get a job? What was it?
28. How did you support yourself?
29. Did you go to school? What was your major?
30. How were your grades, how did you interact with your peers?
31. Did you start doing drugs or alcohol?
32. Did you have any friends, did you have any problems making friends?
33. Did anything significant happen during your adolescence with your parents, siblings, other family members, friends?
34. Did you have a romantic relationship with anyone, how did you meet?
35. Did you have any children? How many and with whom?
36. What was the relationship like with the co-parents?
37. Did anything significant happen during your adulthood with your parents, siblings, other family members, friends? How did you react to this situation?

Middle Adulthood (Ages 31–55)

38. Did you have a job? What was it?
39. How did you support yourself?
40. Are you in a relationship? Did you have any break-ups? How did react to the changes in the relationships?
41. Do you have any children? How old are they? Do they live with you?
42. Did anything significant happen during adulthood with your family? How did you react to this situation?
43. Is there any significant illnesses with you or any significant family members?
44. Are you using any drugs or alcohol? How bad is your use? Did you have to go to rehabilitation?

Late Life (Ages 56+)

45. Did you have a job? What was it?
46. How did you support yourself?
47. Are you in a relationship? Did you have any break-ups? How did react to the changes in the relationships?
48. Do you have any children? How old are they? Do they live with you?
49. Did anything significant happen during adulthood with your family? How did you react to this situation?
50. Are there any significant illnesses with you or any significant family members?
51. Are you using any drugs or alcohol? How bad is your use? Did you have to go to rehabilitation?

A narrative is a story. A narrative is a story. For this assignment, you transform your interview notes into a narrative—that is, a life story—of the colleague you interviewed. You interweave within this narrative an analysis of the life story by applying person and the environment concepts to your understanding and interpretation of that story.

When planning on how best to collect data, it is important to be aware of the practical considerations and best practices for talking with a client such as:

- Determining who you will collect the data from (e.g., the client, friends or family, medical or legal record). There should be multiple sources when collecting data.
- Identify how you will collect the data and how often you will need to access sources to collect the data.
- Establish how you will communicate with people and places you will collect the data. For example, should you act as a person on official business or a down to earth person.
- Protect the privacy and personal information by using carefully controlled procedures for collecting, storing and accessing data that comply with privacy, human rights and other legislation. Dignity and confidentiality must be respected.
- Minimizing the impact and inconvenience of the client when collecting data, which includes choosing the best time to collect the data.
- Aiming for flexibility to allow for changes without great expense or inconvenience.

To collect data about a client's family or a family who is the client. A genogram is useful to collect data (Diagram 7.1).

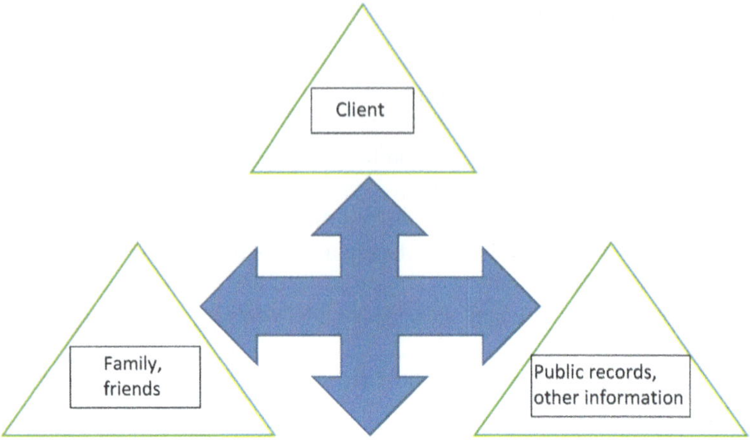

Diagram 7.1 Trifecta of collecting data information

Genogram

A **genogram** (pronounced: *jen-uh-gram*) is a graphic representation of a family tree that displays detailed data on relationships among individuals (Mattaini 1993). It goes beyond a traditional family tree by allowing the worker to analyze hereditary patterns and psychological factors that punctuate relationships. Genograms allows the worker and client to quickly identify and understand various patterns in the patient's family history which may have had an influence on the patient's current state of mind. The genogram maps out relationships and traits that may otherwise be missed on a pedigree chart (Mattaini 1993).

Genograms were first developed and popularized in clinical settings by Monica McGoldrick and Randy Gerson through the publication of a book in 1985. Genograms are now used by various groups of people in a variety of fields such as medicine, psychology, social work, genealogy, genetic research, and education. There are many books and websites on the topic of genograms.

Genograms contain a wealth of information on the families represented. First, they contain basic data found in family trees such as the name, gender, date of birth, and date of death of each individual. Additional data may include education, occupation, major life events, chronic illnesses, social behaviors, nature of family relationships, emotional relationships, and social relationships. Some genograms also include information on disorders running in the family such as alcoholism, depression, diseases, alliances, and living situations. Genograms can vary significantly because there is no limitation as to what type of data can be included (Diagram 7.2).

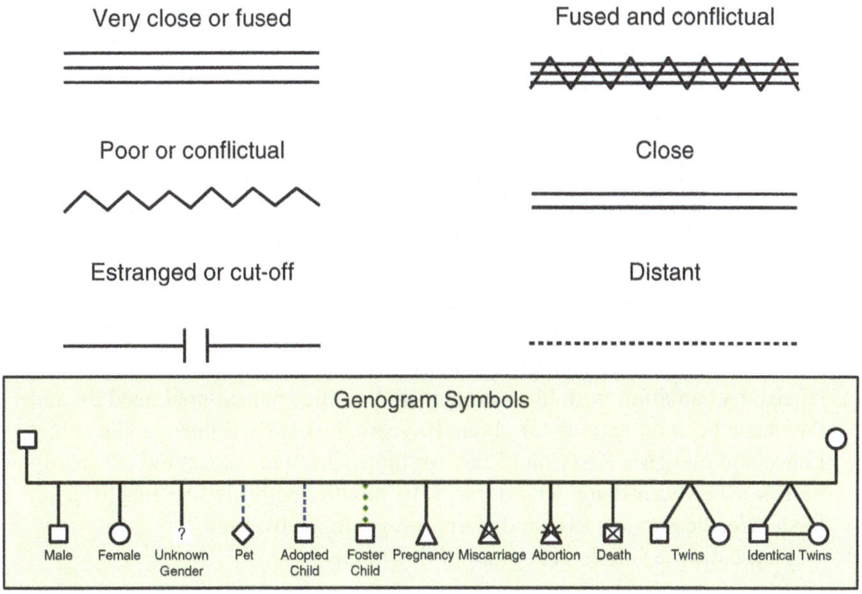

Diagram 7.2 Genogram symbols

Exercise

Case study

Drawing a genogram

Elsa got married at 17 years old to Harry who was 18 years. Her mother Mary, age 80 lives in Brasso Seco and is remarried to Bruce age 87 twenty years ago. Elsa's parents Mary age 80 and Kyle age 86 had six children, Mario, 66; Steve, 60; Sally, 62; Melvin, 59; Elias, 47 and Elsa, 41. Elsa was the last child. Elsa's parents broke up 25 years ago when she was 10 years old and most of her siblings were out of the house. Elsa's father quickly remarried another woman 25 years ago names Cecil age 76. Cecil has two children from a previous marriage to Ben. Cecil and Kyle have no children between the both of them. Elsa's mother and her new husband have no children between them both but Bruce has four children from a previous marriage to Kendra. After her parents' divorced, Elsa and Elias went to live with her mother in Brasso Seco but would visit with her father in Diego Martin on the weekends this is where she met her husband Harry. Harry is one of four children born to

Micheal and Jezelle who were both married. Harry has two brothers, Steve 47; Jeb, 45 and one sister Jewel, 39. Harry's parents have divorced 20 years ago and neither remarried nor had any other children.

Elsa married Harry together they have 5 children. Lance, 23; Elizabeth, 22; Brittany, 21; Sylvia, 19 and Shawna, 16. They have been married for 22 years but within the marriage Harry had multiple extra marital affairs and fathered eight children outside the marriage. There was Sabrina 31 whom he had a 2 year relationship with and fathered a son, Barry aged 12. Then there was Marla 35 who he had a 4 year relationship with and fathered two boys Calvin and Ross aged 10 and 8. Then there was the relationship with Sheena 19 years old, they only lasted 1 year and he father one child angel, 6. It is alleged that he also had an affair with his secretary in the office named noel aged 38 and they have been on and off for about 10 years. It is alleged that she has a boy Lance and two girls Kerry and Lucy for him; 10, 7 and 3 years old. Presently he has a newborn daughter Laura of 10 months with his live in girlfriend Susie. Needless to say Elsa and Harry are getting a divorce.

Please draw a simple genogram of this family.

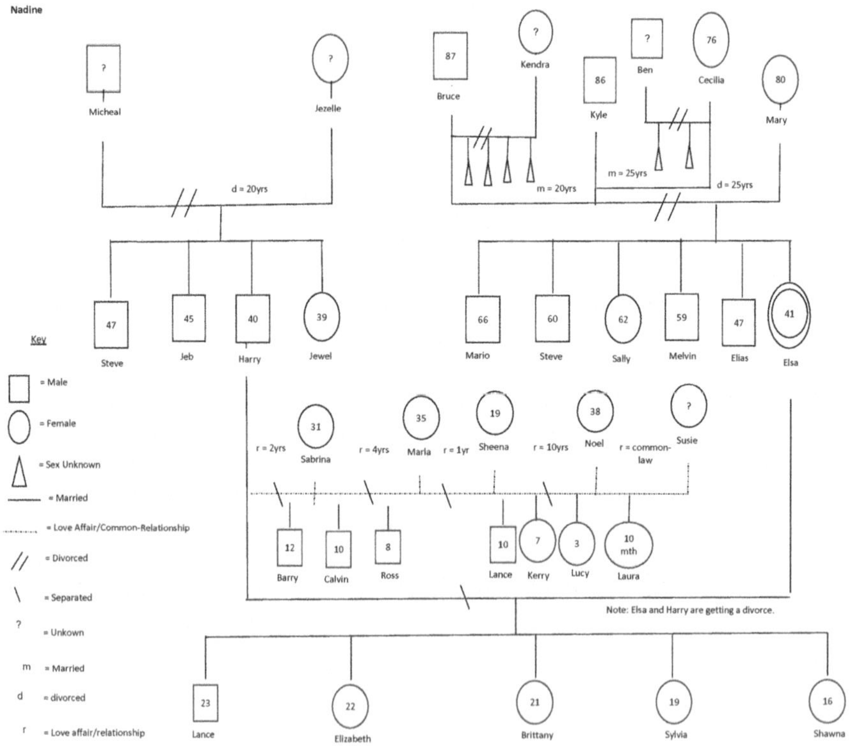

Ecomap

Graphic tools are useful for work on specific types of family issues. An ecological or ecosystems perspective in which clients transactions with environmental systems are taken into account in assessment and intervention. Although many of the graphic tools are techniques considered thus far have substantial utility for realizing this perspective, the ecomap was developed specifically for this purpose. Hartman (1978) discussed the advantages of this simulation tool for assessing and conceptualizing clinical cased holistically and for organizing a large amount of data in a nonlinear contextual fashion. The ecomap is particularly useful for capturing information important to systematic formulations including boundary issues and the direction rate and mutually of resources exchanges while concurrently increasing the client's level involvement in assessment and intervention planning.

Hartman (1978) observed that collaborative use of this tool with clients can dramatically decrease client's defensiveness and that clients often feel the social service worker using it is making a genuine effort to understand their life circumstances. The use of ecomaps reduces the amount of narrative required to capture a case situation, portraying relationships with extended family, formal systems like schools and public welfare offices informal friendship networks and many other relevant factors. It also provides a way of examing each of these factors in the context of the others. Ecomaps are therefore deeply contextual, systemtic tools that are useful for all fields of practice. Hartman suggests that workers keep a supply of blank ecomaps on hand, which can be relatively standardized for a particular setting. Whereas some systems that are commonly salient to cases in the example are listed other circles are left blank to be completed are needed. Specialized ecomaps in which additional detail beyond that commonly found on more standardized ecomaps is provided. Often there are trade-offs between the available time and level of detail so deciding on the extent of individualization and detail to be depicted requires clinical judgment. Hartman (1978) suggests using ecomaps to examine exchanges with systems outside the household and using family mapping separately to examine exchanges within the family. It can be effective to combine the two however to achieve a more integrated picture of the case situation when this can be done without making the image too confusing. The variations in which connections between systems represent relationships- positive, stressful or tenuous and arrows reflect that flow of energy or resources. It is also possible to represent theoretically important exchanges in other ways, such as modelling networks of mutual reinforcement and aversives. Ecomaps have the potential for wide use providing a generic means of modelling and simulating transactional exchanges that define an ecosystems perspective. They can be useful for work at multiple system levels from individual clinical work to community organization and across a broad range of practice approaches. Ecomaps also can be computerized reducing the level of effort required to use them (Diagram 7.3).

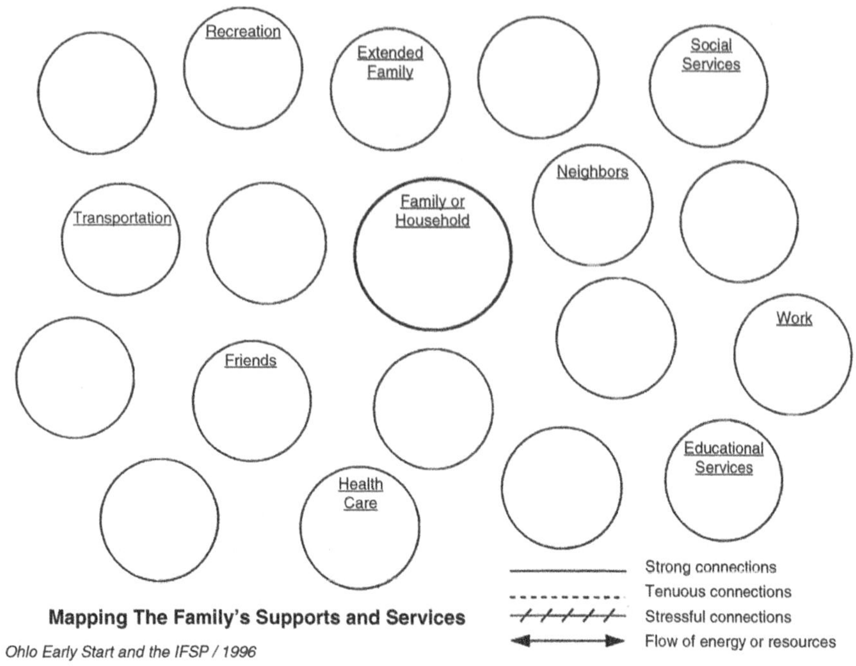

Diagram 7.3 Mapping the family's supports and services

Review Questions

1. In this chapter, there are different methods of collecting data, can you name and describe a few methods of collecting data?
2. Can you describe the different components of the helping interview?
3. How to prepare of an interview using the casework method?
4. Provide a summary of verbal and non-verbal communication.

References

Commiscei. (2017). *Etiquette and taboos: Around the world*. California: Greewood Publishing.

Erikson, E. (1950). *Childhood and society*. New York: W.W. Norton Books.

Freud, S. (1926). Inhibitions, symptoms, and anxiety. In *The standard edition* (Vol. 20). London: Hogarth Press.

Hartman, A. (1978). Diagrammatic assessment of family relationships. *Social Casework, 59*, 465–476.

Johnson, E. J. (2017). An exploratory study on the impact of domestic violence on the families in Trinidad and Tobago, the West Indies. *Journal of Evidence-Informed Social Work, 14*(1), 19–34.

Kirst-Ashman, K., & Hull, G. (2014). *Understanding generalist practice* (7th ed.). Australia: Cernage Learning.

Mattaini, M. (1993). *More than a thousand words: Graphics for clinical practice*. Washington D. C.: National Association of Social Workers.

Chapter 8
Assessment and Intervention

Highlights of this Chapter:

- An overview of the assessment in the casework method.
- An overview of the intervention and termination in the casework method.
- An overview of the Behavior theory for assessment, intervention and termination.
- An overview of the Task-centered approach as a casework method.
- An overview of the problem-solving approach as a casework method.

Assessment

There are different avenues to assess a problem and help a client. There are different therapeutic approaches that should be considered when working with different clients and their problems. The following are three different approaches to assess client's problems and make an accurate social diagnosis. A diagnosis is an explanation based on the facts collected from the client and the client's personality based on a theoretical knowledge base (e.g., Erikson Psychosocial stages of life). The worker is critically analysing the causes such as; the social, environmental, the psychological and personality factors of the problem which brings the client to the worker in the first place. If the problem is a behavioral problem, an eclectic approach to assessing a problem and an accurate assessment of the behavior will help the client access help easier. An eclectic approach means the use of the best of knowledge gathered from a number of different theoretical orientations. Informed eclecticism entails in-depth knowledge of the theoretical approaches from which one selects principles and procedures of action. Taking bits and pieces from many theories and using them casually without any definite purpose is not informed eclecticism (Rengasamy).

E. J. Johnson, C. L. Huggins, *Social Casework Methodology: A Skills Handbook for the Caribbean Human Services Worker*, SpringerBriefs in Social Work,
https://doi.org/10.1007/978-3-030-27319-4_8

The Behavior-Therapy Assessment

Under the behavior assessment the objective is to define as clearly as possible the problem or events based on behavior (e.g., addiction; Thomlison and Thomlison 1996).

1. Gathering of problematic behavior from the client, the family, and other support systems. Clarify the perceived problems by asking for specific behaviors and perception of the problem (see the DSM V, APA 2013).
2. Identify priority behavioral problems, and attempt to identify antecedent events (e.g., traumatic event) that may have triggered the behavior and kept the behavior to continue.
3. Identify the contingencies existent for the provision of consequences.
4. Identify recurrent behavior patterns.
5. Secure a commitment from all members of the family system or support systems who wish to work toward change in the client.
6. Begin to identify possible behavior target for change.
7. Discuss possible appropriate behavioral targets for change. Select behavior that are to be increased in frequency in order to maximize the opportunities for positive consequences. Select and review behaviors that are incompatible with problematic behaviors.
8. Allow time for the clients and their support systems (e.g. family).
9. When target behaviors have been agreed upon, set the conditions for a baseline measure. Before instructing the client to change, request that the behaviors are monitored for frequency of occurance of the target behaviors.
10. During the assessment phase, a behavioral intervention is necessary with an assessment in progress to help the client concentrate on the couple's problems.

The behavior theory assessment only targets behaviors and may neglect other issues such as, environmental stressors. It is best when this assessment approach be used in tandem with other assessment frameworks that deal with other issues such as the environment.

Problem-Solving Framework Assessment

Another assessment framework that can be used to diagnose problems and help clients is a problem-solving framework which is a cognitive activity aimed at changing a problem to a goal (Mayer 1994). Problem solving shares with psychodynamic theory a belief in the necessity for an empathic, caring, supporting, enhancing type of relationship and acknowledges that such as approach works particularly well with clients who are trusting, responsive to warmth and able to reach out for help when needed. The problem-solving approach is also able to respond to and engage the resistant and nonvoluntary client and the natural ambivalence that occurs with negative feelings arise or when expectations are not fully met.

It is a systematic, step by step thinking process moving from an undesired to a desired state (Gerlfand 1988). Problem-solving theory is a direct practice theory for working with individuals, couples, families and groups. Problem solving draws a conceptual map to guide both workers and clients through the stages and steps involved in a change process designed to move from the problem to the solution. Problem solving is nicely aligned with casework method because problem solving draws a conceptual map to guide both the client and the worker through the stages and steps involved in a change process designed to move the client from the problem to the solution (Turner and Jaco 1996). The problem-solving framework is linear as well as circular in nature in any of the stages, which means stages loop back to an earlier stage or forward to a step that lies in the future, if the circumstances require it. Perlman (1957) saw living as a problem-solving process and she described life as a continuous change and movement in which the human being works on so adapting himself to external objects to achieve maximum satisfaction.

Behavior therapy provides a planned systematic approach to the casework method. The goal of behavioral therapy are to increase desirable behaviors and reduce undesirable behaviors in order that the client can improve daily functioning. The basic behavioral assessment method is used to analyze the client's problem and assist in a plan of change by developing appropriate behavioral change goals. The process is flexible in nature, allowing considerable latitude in its application. The problem-solving assessment model (Turner and Jaco 1996):

1. Contact phase
   a. Problem identification- as seen by client, others, and worker. Problem for work identified,
   b. Goal identification- short and long term goals stated. What does the client wish for or need. What resources are available?
   c. Contract- preliminary in nature as it consists of clarifying the agency's resources and committing to further study of the problem.
   d. Exploration- of the client's motivation, opportunities and capacities.
2. Contract Phase
   a. Assessment and evaluation
      i. How are problems related to needs of client systems?
      ii. What factors contribute to creating and maintaining of the problem?
      iii. What resources and strengths does the client have?
      iv. What knowledge and principles could be applied from theoretical perspectives?

One of the difficulties in applying a problem-solving assessment to real life situations is that it is too challenging to process all of the information called for in the various stages (Osmo and Rosen 1994) and as a consequence, people choose the solution that best satisfies their needs in the short term although it may be far from optimal. Other problems related to problem solving are the following:

1. Lack of clarity in stating the problem, this step requires time as the process is bound to fail.
2. Not getting the needed information; minimal information results in poor problem definition, fewer alternative strategies with consequence inaccurately predicted.
3. Poor communication among those involved in the process, communication is central to the entire method from definition to task allocation so clarity and comprehensiveness must remain goals of the interchange.
4. Premature testing of alternative strategies; the process discourages creative thinking and free expression, a direction which has not been thoroughly discussed might be chosen.
5. Climate in which decisions are made is critical or demands conformity.
6. Lack of skills in problem-solving; people can be trained to use the method in the context of their current problem.
7. Motivation is lacking, people who problem solve must have some need to change their situation and hope that it can be changed. Pressure to change may come from many sources but the experience of engaging in the process itself can generate hope.

Task-Centered Assessment Process

The last assessment framework is the task-centered assessment process. The task centered model is a brief psychological casework method that is efficient to help individuals and families with problems in the family relations. The task-centered approach is time limited and short term in its assessment of problems (Reid 1996). The focus of services is on specific problems clients explicitly acknowledge as being of concern to the client.

The client-worker relationship is a caring but collaborative effort to avoid hidden goals and agenda; extensive use is made of client's input in developing treatment strategies not only to devise more effective interventions, but to develop the client's problem-solving abilities (Reid 1996). Problems are explored and clarified by the worker and the client in the initial interview. The focus is on what the client wants and not on what the worker thinks the client may need. The worker may however point out potential difficulties that the client does not mention. In other words the target problem is not necessarily defined by what clients say they want initially but rather by what they want after a process of deliberation to which workers contribute their own knowledge and point of view. As a result, clients may alter their perception of their problems or in the case of involuntary clients may realize they have difficulties they may wish to work on. At the end of this process, normally at the close of the first or second interview, the worker and client must come to an explicit agreement on the problem(s) to be dealt with (Reid 1996).

Problem exploration is the data-gathering tool for assessing activities, which involve efforts to understand the dynamics of the problem and its contextual features as well as to delineate the frequency and severity of its occurrence (Reid 1996). A largely cognitive process, assessment is led by the worker but should also involve the client as collaborator. While the worker can contribute professional knowledge, the client has unique personal knowledge of the problem and its context. Assessment is essentially problem-focused. It starts with the problems to be dealt with and incorporate whatever information about the client's situation, such as history, personality that might be relevant to those problems (Reid 1996).

In exploring and assessing problems, workers may make use of a variety of theories (e.g., systems theory, Maslow's hierarchy of needs) depending on what best fits the problem at hand. In the task-centered model, problems are derived empirically from client's view of their difficulties as these are clarified in interviews with the worker. Workers do not use theory to formulate problems but rather start with a description of the problem and then scan relevant knowledge, including theories to locate possible explanations for the issue. Certain guidelines are offered for this theory: whatever hypotheses are selected to explain the problem should be evaluated through case data (Reid 1996). This involves analysing evidence to determine the likelihood of the hypothesis holding in the particular case. Preference is given to theories that have been supported by empirical research (Reid 1996). The worker does not fixate on a single explanation but rather considers alternative explanations in a search for the theory that provides the best fit with the problem and the case at hand.

The worker and client develop a contract in which the client agrees to work with the worker on one or more problem(s). The worker and client develop a rationale or purpose for carrying out the task if it is not already clear. Either the worker or the client might first consider the potential benefit to be gained from completing the task. During the process the client's progress on resolving the problem and the tasks are routinely reviewed at the beginning of each interview (Reid 1996). The review covers developments in the problem and what the client has and has not accomplished in tasks to resolve it. The worker reviews their tasks in a similar manner. What the worker does next depends on the results of the review and if the tasks have been substantially accomplished or completed, the worker may formulate another task with the client on the same problem or a different problem (Reid 1996). If the task has not been carried out or only partially achieved, the worker and client may discuss obstacles. Devise a different plan for carrying out the task. The task may be revised or replaced by another task.

The preceding assessment models (e.g., behavioral therapy assessment, problem solving theory assessment and task-centred assessment model) are just a few assessment models that can be used in the casework method. They are all effective and evidence-based and can be used as an eclectic approach when helping clients. Next is the intervention process and treatment for the problems utilizing the same models of behavior therapy, problem-solving theory and task-cantered models.

Intervention/Treatment

A wide range of interventions exist that address a variety of problems. Many of these interventions target behaviors (e.g., depressive symptoms). Other interventions target a specific problem, such as disruptive behaviors in dementia, or pain in patients with cancer. Careful assessment need to be completed before implementing any of these interventions because the focus of the intervention needs to address the particular needs of the client. For many of these clinical approaches, building skills in coping, problem-solving, increasing the rate of pleasant activity for the client are either the explicit goal of interventions or are the active ingredient in the interventions prescribed.

Behavior Therapy – Intervention

The behavior therapy – intervention is marked by the identification of new possibilities that might occur between identified behaviors and the consequences of these behaviors. The sequence of the behaviors are (Thomlison and Thomlison 1996):

1. Clarify and identify the target behaviors that are the focus for change.
2. Establish a new trigger for each of the targeted new behaviors.
3. Establish new consequences that are to be provided for each occurrence or non-occurrence of a targeted behavior.
4. Formulate a contract with the client: target behaviors for change; new positive consequences for behavior change; specify what is to happen if there is a violation of the contract that is if an undesired behavior occurs.
5. It is necessary to follow up with a series of telephone calls to ensure that the program has been implemented.
6. Difficulties in implementing the program are inevitable. These problems usually pertain to such things as tally recording, difference in target behavior definition and lack of cooperation on the part of certain family member.
7. Each interview with the client and family after implementation should begin with an examination of the tally recording provided by family member.
8. Discussion must then shift to problems arising between sessions. If family members are involved the worker must spend time on areas in the family life. One of the advantages of having required that family to negotiate changes in the behavior.

Problem-Solving Approach: Intervention

The problem-solving approach for intervention and treatment. The problem-solving process is good for clients who come for help only when they feel that a crisis exists and the emphasis is on the here and now. Problem-solving therapy is a present centered, reality-based model of practice that focuses on where the client is at the crucial time of needing and seeking out help (Turner and Jaco 1996). It expects that persons have an ability to work toward both solving their problems and using their powers to bring about new experiences both rewarding and fulfilling in terms of an increased competence to handle the problems of everyday life. A major component of the assessment in problem solving is to focus on the present as well as it acknowledgment of the power of the therapeutic relationship to motivate and engage the client in working on the identified problem.

Formulation of a plan of action.

i. Set reachable goals.
ii. Examine alternatives and their likely outcomes.
iii. Determine appropriate method of service
iv. Identify focus of change efforts.
v. Clarify roles of work and client.

a. Prognosis-What is worker's hope for success.

Action Phase

1. Carrying out the plan.
   i. Specify point of intervention and assign tasks.
   ii. Identify resources and services to be used.
   iii. Indicate who is to do what and when.

The original focus of intervention was the person's inability to cope with a problem due to some lack of motivation or opportunity. Underlying the approach was the basic assumption that all of human living involves satisfaction rather than frustration and punishment. A strong relationship between education and therapy and promote a person's confidence and gratification in the client ability to employ problem-solving strategies in a helpful manner. It was acknowledged that education is chiefly addressed to intellectual abilities and therapy to motivational drives and directions, casework was seen as being halfway between education and therapy.

Task-Centered Approach

During the intervention stage of task-centered approach the concentration of obstacles to task achievement and problem change are usually encountered. The target problem is a difficulty standing in a way of progress toward resolution of a target problem and an obstacle is that the former is a difficulty that the client and the worker have contracted to change. Obstacles block progress, resources facilitate it. Resources are usually found in strengths and competencies of individual clients, in the ties of loyalty and affection that hold families together and in the intangible and tangible support provided by external systems (Reid 1996). A characteristic may serve as either an obstacle or resource depending on its function in relation to the problem. The worker helps clients to identify and resolve obstacles as well as to locate and utilize resources. The discussion is led by the worker who relies on focused exploration, explanations, and other methods designed to increase the client's understanding. The process may overlap with the problem and task assessment when obstacles and resources may emerge and be explored (Reid 1996). The worker may help clients modify distorted perceptions or unrealistic expectations. Dysfunctional patterns of behavior or interactions may be pointed out (Johnson 2018).

Evaluation-Termination

Evaluation is a continual process throughout the contact, were the purposes accomplished, were appropriate methods chosen to induce change, what has client learned that can be used in ongoing problem solving, what can worker learn to help with similar cases.

Behavior Theory Termination- Evaluation (Thomlison and Thomlison 1996).

1. Monitor the change to indicate that little if any change is taking place, it is necessary to examine certain aspects of the program design.
2. When target behaviors have been achieved at the desired level of frequency identify new behaviors for change or move toward termination.
3. Together with the client evaluate progress in relation to the objectives of the contact.
4. If the decision is to terminate, set the conditions for behavioral maintenance.
5. Behavioral maintenance requires the worker to review with the family the basic learning principles identified during the modification of the target behavior.
6. Instruct the family to continue the tally recording over the next 4 weeks but without the regularly scheduled appointments.
7. Set up an appointment for 4 weeks from the last interview for the purposes of termination and follow-up.

The follow-up interview should assess whether or not the behavoral changes have been maintained. If they have not been maintained at the level consistent with the expectations of the worker, it will be necessary to reinstitute the program structure. From the perspective of clinical evaluation it is important that the worker analyze the results of the behavioral change program. Further it is helpful for the worker to contact clients at three and 6 month intervals to ascertain the degree to which the behavioral changes have been maintained.

Together with the family system evaluate in relation to the objectives of the contract. If the decision is to terminate, set the conditions for behavioral maintenance (Thomlison and Thomlison 1996).

Behavioral maintenance requires the social worker to review with the family the basic learning principles identified during the modification of the target behvavior (e.g., positive consequences vs. punishment).

Insruct the family to continue the tally recording over the next 4 weeks but without the regularly scheduled appointments. Set up an appointment for 4 weeks from the last interview for the purposes of termination and follow-up.

The follow-up interview should assess whether or not the behavioral changes have been maintained. If they have not been maintained at a level consistent with the expectations of the worker and /or the family. It will be necessary to reinstitute the program structure. If on the other hand, the worker and family feel that the behavioral changes have been maintained within desired parameters, termination may take place. Termination of course does allow for the family to contact the worker at any point in the future when they feel the necessity. From the perspective of a clinical evaluation, it is important that the worker analyze the results of the behavioral change program (Thomlison and Thomlison 1996). Further it is helpful for the worker to contact family members at 3 months and 6 months intervals to ascertain the degree to which the behavioral changes have been maintained.

Problem-Solving Approach: Termination

Evaluate with client system accomplishments and their meaning, learn with client about reasons for lack of success, talk about ways to maintain gains, cope with ending of relationship, review supports in natural network (Compton and Galaway 1994). A continual process throughout contact, purposes accomplished, appropriate methods chosen to induce change, what has the client learned that can be used in ongoing problem solving, what can worker, learn to help with similar cases.

Evaluation a continual process throughout contact, were purposes accomplished. Were appropriate methods chosen to induce change. What has client learned that can be used in ongoing problem solving. What can worker learn to help with similar cases.

The complete models from contract, assessment, termination and evaluation.

Task-Centered Termination

The process of terminating begun in the initial phase when the duration of treatment is set. The worker and client have worked continuously on tasks to resolve the problem and develop new ones that might undertake on their own. What the client has achieved is given stress (Reid 1996). Extensions usually involve a small number of additional sessions, in only a minority of cases in most settings beyond agreed upon time limits are normally made if the client request additional service.

When the task centered system is used in full as the sole of primary method of treatment, its range of applications, is broad enough to serve as a basic approach for the majority of clients seen by workers, it is possible to identify certain types of clients for whom the model in full may not provide the optimal mode of practice. Such types would include the following (Reid 1996): (1). Clients who are not interested in taking action to solve specific problems in their life situation but who rather want help in exploring existential issues such as concerns about life goals or identity or who wish to talk about stressful experiences. (2). Clients who are unwilling or unable to utilize the structure of the model. (3). Clients who wish to alter conditions, such as certain psychogenic and motor difficulties for which it is not possible to identify problem-solving tasks that the client is able to carry out. (4). Clients who wish no help but may need to be seen for proactive reasons.

Behavior Theory Approach (Thomlison and Thomlison 1996)

Gathering of problematic behavior from the client, the family, and other support systems. Clarify the perceived problems by asking for specific behaviors and perception of the problem (see the DSM V, APA 2013).

1. Identify priority behavioral problems, and attempt to identify antecedent events (e.g., traumatic event) that may have triggered the behavior and kept the behavior to continue.
2. Identify the contingencies existent for the provision of consequences.
3. Identify recurrent behavior patterns.
4. Secure a commitment from all members of the family system or support systems who wish to work toward change in the client.
5. Begin to identify possible behavior target for change.
6. Discuss possible appropriate behavioral targets for change. Select that are to be increased in frequency in order to maximize the opportunities for positive consequences. Select and review behaviors that are incompatible with problematic behaviors.
7. Allow time for the clients and their support systems (e.g. family).
8. When target behaviors have been agreed upon, set the conditions for a baseline measure. Before instructing the client to change, request that the behaviors are monitored for frequency of occurrence of the target behaviors.
9. During the assessment phase, a behavioral intervention is necessary with an assessment in progress to help the client concentrate on the couple's problems.
10. Clarify and identify the target behaviors that are the focus for change.
11. Establish a new trigger for each of the targeted new behaviors.
12. Establish new consequences that are to be provided for each occurrence or non-occurrence of a targeted behavior.
13. Formulate a contract with the client: target behaviors for change; new positive consequences for behavior change; specify what is to happen if there is a violation of the contract that is if an undesired behavior occurs.
14. It is necessary to follow up with a series of telephone calls to ensure that the program has been implemented.
15. Difficulties in implementing the program are inevitable. These problems usually pertain to such things as tally recording, difference in target behavior definition and lack of cooperation on the part of certain family member.

16. Each interview with the client and family after implementation should begin with an examination of the tally recording provided by family member.
17. Discussion must then shift to problems arising between sessions. If family members are involved the worker must spend time on areas in the family life. One of the advantages of having required that family to negotiate changes in the behavior.
18. Monitor the change to indicate that little if any change is taking place, it is necessary to examine certain aspects of the program design.
19. When target behaviors have been achieved at the desired level of frequency identify new behaviors for change or move toward termination.
20. Together with the client evaluate progress in relation to the objectives of the contact.
21. If the decision is to terminate, set the conditions for behavioral maintenance.
22. Behavioral maintenance requires the worker to review with the family the basic learning principles identified during the modification of the target behavior.
23. Instruct the family to continue the tally recording over the next 4 weeks but without the regularly scheduled appointments.
24. Set up an appointment for 4 weeks from the last interview for the purposes of termination and follow-up.

The follow-up interview should assess whether the behavioral changes have been maintained. If they have not been maintained at the level consistent with the expectations of the worker, it will be necessary to reinstitute the program structure. From the perspective of clinical evaluation, it is important that the worker analyze the results of the behavioral change program. Further it is helpful for the worker to contact clients at three and six-month intervals to ascertain the degree to which the behavioral changes have been maintained.

The problem-solving model (Turner and Jaco 1996):

1. Contact phase

   a. Problem identification- as seen by client, others, and worker. Problem for work identified,
   b. Goal identification- short and long term goals stated. What does the client wish for or need. What resources are available?
   c. Contract- preliminary in nature as it consists of clarifying the agency's resources and committing to further study of the problem.
   d. Exploration- of the client's motivation, opportunities and capacities.

2. Contract Phase

   e. Assessment and evaluation

      i. How are problems related to needs of client systems?
      ii. What factors contribute to creating and maintaining of the problem?
      iii. What resources and strengths does the client have?
      iv. What knowledge and principles could be applied from theoretical perspectives?

Other problems related to problem solving are the following:

1. Lack of clarity in stating the problem, this step requires time as the process is bound to fail.
2. Not getting the needed information; minimal information results in poor problem definition, fewer alternative strategies with consequence inaccurately predicted.
3. Poor communication among those involved in the process, communication is central to the entire method from definition to task allocation so clarity and comprehensiveness must remain goals of the interchange.
4. Premature testing of alternative strategies; the process discourages creative thinking and free expression, a direction which has not been thoroughly discussed might be chosen.
5. Climate in which decisions are made is critical or demands conformity.
6. Lack of skills in problem-solving; people can be trained to use the method in the context of their current problem.
7. Motivation is lacking, people who problem solve must have some need to change their situation and hope that it can be changed. Pressure to change may come from many sources but the experience of engaging in the process itself can generate hope.

Formulation of a plan of action.

v. Set reachable goals.
vi. Examine alternatives and their likely outcomes.
vii. Determine appropriate method of service
viii. Identify focus of change efforts.
ix. Clarify roles of work and client.

a. Prognosis-What is worker's hope for success.

Action Phase

b. Carrying out the plan.

x. Specify point of intervention and assign tasks.
xi. Identify resources and services to be used.
xii. Indicate who is to do what and when.

Termination

Evaluate with client system accomplishments and their meaning, learn with client about reasons for lack of success, talk about ways to maintain gains, cope with ending of relationship, review supports in natural network. A continual process throughout contact, purposes accomplished, appropriate methods chosen to induce change, what has the client learned that can be used in ongoing problem solving, what can worker, learn to help with similar cases.

Evaluation a continual process throughout contact, were purposes accomplished. Were appropriate methods chosen to induce change. What has client learned that can be used in ongoing problem solving. What can worker learn to help with similar cases.

The complete models from contract, assessment, termination and evaluation.

Review Questions

1. In this chapter, there are three methods for assessment, intervention and termination, can you name and describe one approach?
2. Can you describe what is the assessment, intervention and termination in the casework method?

Case Studies

Each case study is set in Caribbean, please read each case study and answer the attached questions.

Valerie

Valerie is a 69 year-old woman of mixed ethnicity (Spanish and an African) who has sole custody of 14 year old Avery, her grandson. Events leading up to this arrangement was that her son Paul at 16 years old attending Caribbean Union College met Rose a 16 year old girl who already had a 2 year old son at the time at a party and soon after Rose gave birth to Avery. At 17 years old Paul dropped out of school and found a job to support his newborn son and Rose. All of them initially lived with Valerie and eventually moved out to an apartment in Tacarigua. After 3 months Paul felt the rent was too expensive and decided to move back in with his mother Valerie.

Valerie not knowing much about Rose other than she was a very small young girl with long black hair and dull yellow eyes was quite surprised with Rose passed away when Avery was 11 months old. The cause of death according to the corner was a rare form of renal failure. Paul, Valerie's son was devastated by this and left Avery in the care of her while he pursued his business interests. Shortly thereafter, Paul became a small business owner where he sold items like clothing, perfumes and shoes on the pavement in Arima. He was successful for 3 years until he was shot twice in the arm and once in the stomach while seated in his car. Avery was 5 years old. Valerie recalls she was a passenger in a maxi taxi on her way to work when she received a call from her daughter that Paul has been shot. She recalls screaming murder and for someone to help her. When Valerie arrived to the Arima Health facility she saw her son's corpse wrapped in a white sheet. Approximately 1 year after the death of Paul, Valerie sought legal guardianship of Avery and has been caring for him ever since.

At 8 years old Avery is about 4 feet 11″ and about 120 pounds, he is slightly taller than other children and maintains a serious face most of the time. According to Valerie, Avery is always upset about something. At home Avery is unable to sit still for long periods of time. He also pushes his younger cousins around since he is the oldest grandchild. Avery is a confident child with good eye contact and expressive language skills, he has healthy skin and nails.

Valerie states she has a great relationship with Avery, he is helpful in the kitchen and carrying out duties around the house. Avery is generally respectful to adults but at times he is rude and disrespectful to his aunts and Valerie's present husband. Avery also has an uncle who beats him using his hands, feet, spoons, a dog leash, stones or anything he gets his hands on. Sometimes he is left with scars. Also when he is rude, Avery is physically punished and made to kneel for approximately 2–3 hrs on the tiled floor. He is also hit on his knuckles, knees and shin with a hairbrush.

In form one Avery's behavior was described as acceptable in the first -term and then in the second term teachers started complaining that Avery was bullying other students, fighting often and stealing other children's items. Avery is only disrespectful and will curse other children if they are disrespectful to him and talk about his mother offensively. Avery is usually pays attention in class except for Math and science. Although he like Mathematics his math teacher once called him, "filthy" and he did not like her comment so he refuses to pay attention in her class. In form two, the teachers claim Avery is intelligent but will fight other student and is sometimes disrespectful however he has never been suspended from school. The teachers also claim Avery does not have difficulty understanding any subjects and can apply himself to anything.

Avery indicated that he first learned that his father died when he was only 8 years old and his first thought was "no more licks". Avery did not cry at the funeral and misses his father a lot when he thinks about him. Avery stated he does not miss his mother because he never knew her and his grandmother fills the role of mom in his life.

Questions

1. Who is the client?
2. What is the presenting problem?
3. What casework approach would you use for this case and why?

Rhonda

Rhonda is a 28 year old East Indian woman who presented her 7 year old daughter Carrie to the Child Guidance Clinic in Port of Spain regarding a recent incident that occurred with her brother Ismeal who is 20 years old.

Rhonda stated her family history where her mother Olivia left the family home when Rhonda was 12 years old. Rhonda lived with her father and siblings Ismeal (20), Calvin (25) and Silva (26). Rhonda's paternal grandmother lived in the same house and assisted with raising the children when her father went to work. Rhonda indicated that she had to look after her younger siblings and assumed all the household duties (i.e., cleaning, cooking, washing) after her mother left the home, she was 13 years old. At the age of 14, Rhonda and her siblings was taken by her father to live with his girlfriend in Sangre Grande for a few months to be closer to her school. Rhonda stated she dropped out of school in Form 1 because of lack of family support. She sold cigarettes and braided hair in order to support herself. At age 15, Rhonda went to live with her mother and Raj, live-in boyfriend in Arima. She lived there for approximately 2 years. She states she has had a rocky relationship with her mother but got along with her boyfriend. At age 16, Rhonda met Lin who was Raj's friend and started a visiting relationship.

Lin was living with his mother and she moved in with them at the age of 17. Rhonda and Lin had Carrie and a little baby boy Kazam and Rhonda has been living with Lin ever since. Lin financially cares for the family and Rhonda maintains the housekeeping. On November 2013, Rhonda was home with her baby son and Carrie when her brother Ismeal arrived at her home about 9 am. This was not uncommon as he would visit their home approximately twice a week to have his hair braided. Ismeal would occasionally sleep on the couch in the living room. That day Ismeal was looking upkept and Rhonda told him to take a bath and change his clothes. After Ismeal took his bath Rhonda asked him to hold the baby while she also took a bath. The bathroom was located outside the house. When Rhonda returned Carrie told her ismeal pulled down his pants and touched her vagina, anus and put his penis in her mouth and told her to "lick it".

Horrified Rhonda went to the neighbour's house and contacted the police and Lin. When the police arrived Ismeal admitted that he placed his penis in Carrie's mouth. Ismeal pleaded with her and told her that a male neighbour has incestuous relations with him when he was 8 years old. Ismeal was then handcuffed and taken to the police station. Statements were taken and the police said that it didn't look like anything happened to Carrie. Carrie was not examined at that time. Rhonda looked at her brother and saw he was very remorseful and decided to drop the charges. Ismeal never visited Rhonda again and his father bailed him out of jail and no charges were pressed. Since then there has been no other occurrence of sexual abuse.

When Rhonda arrived home and went to give Carrie a bathe, she noticed that Carrie stated it her vagina and anus was burning her and she was unable to take a bowel movement for approximately 2 weeks due to the burning sensation. Carrie was examined by My. Hope and the blood work confirmed everything was normal and the examination did not confirm there was penetration.

Since the incident Carrie has become hyperactive and at times been screaming and shouting in school and at home. Carrie has regressed at school and in one incident removed her underwear and pant and threw it over the fence and even urinated behind the school. Carrie is restless, refusing to stay in her seat and has trouble sleeping at night. Carrie also has a low appetite. Rhonda has also been depressed and unable to function at home with her chores for at least 3 months. Rhonda also indicated that Lin is no longer affectionate towards her and they have not had any intercourse for approximately 2–3 month after the incident took place

Questions

1. Who is the client?
2. What is the presenting problem?
3. What casework approach would you use for this case and why?
4. Create three questions you would use during the interview.

Tammy

Tammy is a 16 year old female of Indian and an African descent who was referred to the Child Guidance Clinci by the Eric William Medical Science complex regarding concerns of being raped, using obsene language, destroying property, attempted homicide of her mother and suicide. She a pretty well-kept young lady, who is slender with broad shoulder, her is a jet black and shoulder length.

Tammy was born to Cheryl and Horace in 1997. The Parent met in 1991 and maintained a visiting relationship, they had a miscarriage in May 1997 and Cheryl was pregnant with Tammy in 1997. In 1998, the couple ended the relationship because Horace was Anglican and wanted Tammy to be baptized as an Anglican and Cheryl was Roman Catholic and wanted Tammy to be baptized Roman Catholic. Horace also wanted his friends to be Tammy's God parents and Cheryl objected to the notion. The couple relationship was rekindled in 1999 but ended in 2002 when Horace became involved in another relationship. Horace maintained a relationship with his daughter until she was 11 years old. Tammy complained that when she visited with her father he was often engaged in a sexual relationship with his girlfriend and would send her outside in the yard. Tammy also complained that he did not spend any quality time with her and his girlfriend often interfered in their conversations so Tammy no longer wanted to visit with him.

Cheryl met Morris in 2002 and they started a visiting relationship and gave birth to a boy Rowan. Tammy and Morris had a decent relationship as he was involved in her life. The couple ended their relationship in 2009. In 2011 Cheryl met and married Clarence and they all have been living together ever since.

In 2012 Tammy started going to MOMS and Cheryl hired a driver to take her to and from school. One morning in January Tammy told the driver to take her home so she could change her t-shirt. Tammy stated that when she went into her bedroom in her bra the driver threw her on the bed and began to kiss her. Then he took her back to school. Sometime again in April Tammy went back to the driver's house where the driver attempted to have sexual intercourse with Tammy. He did not succeed and he took her back to school. At the time Tammy never told anyone about the incident, but later that month she tried to hang herself at her home. According to Cheryl, Tammy stood on the window ledge, tied a piece of rope around the burglar proof bar, tied a piece of rope around her neck and was about to jump when her maternal grandmother and stepfather stopped her.

Tammy complained to her family that no one loves her. A week later she was washing dishes and started to cry uncontrollably. When Cheryl approached her to find out what was wrong she told her that the driver attempted to rape her. The mother immediately took Tammy to the police station and reported the incident and Tammy was examined at the San Juan Health Center. Tammy was also referred for counselling and complained to the counsellor that she was seeing dead people. Tammy was then warded at Eric Williams Medical Complex and spent 1 week.

In 2013, Tammy began attending Eternal Life Vocational School. A couple of months later Tammy became physically and verbally aggressive to mother, younger sibling, stepfather, maternal aunt and maternal grandmother. She threatened her family with knives, used obscene language in the home and in public. To date Tammy continues to threaten her family. In one incident the family went on a boat ride and it is alleged that Kerwin, Morris's friend and 35 years old gave an alcoholic drink to Tammy without getting the parents' permission. When the parents found out about the incident more information was revealed that Tammy has been seen in Kerwin's car on several occasions. When Cheryl confronted Tammy, Tammy denied there was a relationship going on.

Starting 2014, Tammy went to purchase a loaf of bread and did not return home for at least 2 h. When Cheryl called her cell phone, Tammy did not answer. After 3 h Tammy returned home and ran to the bathroom to take a shower. Her maternal grandmother when to check on her and saw there was a bite mark on one of her breasts and a bruise mark on her back. When prompted to find out what happened, Tammy refused to talk to her mother. Tammy however did tell one of her mother's friends that she got into a fight with three men. When Cheryl found out this information, she took Tammy to the police station and made a report.

During Carnival time Cheryl took the children to see the festivities and saw her ex-boyfriend Morris who was working as a security guard. When Tammy saw him he was talking to another woman and she got upset. Tammy began to argue with Morris and accused him of having sex with her. Morris was arrested and is currently incarcerated. Later in March Tammy began to complain of stomach pains and her mother took her to the hospital. The doctor told her Tammy was pregnant. Cheryl asked the police officer what she should do about Tammy and the police officer said do what is necessary. Upon leaving the hospital Cheryl went to the pharmacy and purchased Cyotec. When they arrived home Cheryl inserted the Cyotec into Tammy's vagina and Tammy bled for 8 days. Tammy ultimately miscarried.

Since this incident Tammy states that her sleeping patterns have been affected and was prescribed sleeping pills. Tammy took the sleeping pills and crushed them in a jug of juice and placed it in the refrigerator. Clarence, her step father poured some of the juice in a glass tasted it and found that it tasted funny. Later the family found out Tammy placed the sleeping tablets in the jug. The family did not report the incident. In June, 2014 Cheryl was sitting in her bedroom when Tammy came behind her and tied a rope and a piece of twine around her neck, Tammy began to tighten the rope and twine while accusing Cheryl of taking a piece of paper that belonged to her. According the Tammy's maternal grandmother the paper in question was all the information about Tammy's sexual activities such as the days and nights Tammy left the house without permission. The grandmother pulled Tammy off her Cheryl and Cheryl ran to a neighbour's house.

Questions

1. Who is the client?
2. What is the presenting problem?
3. What casework approach would you use for this case and why?
4. Create three questions you would use during the interview.

Ms. Wallis

Ms. Wallis is a 60 year, an African female old retired cleaner from the QRC secondary school she appears 10 years younger than her stated age. She is alert, oriented time three and able to make her needs known. She has an inviting smile and very talkative. She is a practicing roman catholic and attends church on Sundays and wears a picture of the saints on a necklace for protection. She was referred to the Eric Williams Medical Science Complex medical unit social service department regarding her son.

She complains of sleepless nights and restlessness. Her prior medical history was a surgery for fibroids in the early 1990's as a result of heavy menstruation and benign lumps in her breast. She has a history of high blood pressure and cholesterol. She states her family has had a history of mental illness starting with her sister who was diagnosed with schizophrenia when she was 20 years old. Ms. Wallis stated she is originally from St. Kitts but migrated with her family to Trinidad when she was very young. Her father came to Trinidad seeking employment and more opportunities in Trinidad. Her father worked for the Trinidad and Tobago electric company and died unexpectedly in 1977 due to alleged food poisoning. Her mother was a cleaner at the then Polytechnic college renamed University of Trinidad and Tobago. Her mother also went to college and obtained a bachelor's degree in food and nutrition. Her mother later worked for the General hospital in Port of Spain as a dietician for 30 years. When her mother fell ill Ms. Wallis was her caregiver.

Ms. Wallis states that she was sickly as a child with cold and asthma and was absent from school a lot. She did finish 5 years of secondary education but was not successful at siting for the General Counsil Examinations. From then she was supported by her mother and attended courses for sewing. She met and married Fitzroy and 1 year into the marriage she had a son named Maxwell. Fitzroy migrated to England to study and she was to join him shortly. As her mother had a stroke and she cared for her, Ms. Wallis plans to migrate was curtailed and her marriage eventually ended. When Ms. Wallis' mother passed, she was in her 30's and did not have much work experience. Ms. Wallis younger sister was also living with her and she suddenly passed away in the house. Her sister had her first mental breakdown 1 year after having a baby out of wedlock. Her sister's cause of death was elileptic seizure asphyxiation. She was 39.

Ms. Wallis has a live in relationship with George who is 5 years younger than her. Ms. Wallis has her pension and receives a disability cheque of $1500tt for her son. George works periodically as a security guard in Port of Spain.

Ms. Wallis states when Maxwell was 16 years old he was diagnosed with schizophrenia. At 34 years old he is now incapacitated and needs constant care. Maxwell does not have control of his bodily functions and wears a diaper. Maxwell often does not like to take a shower and when he does it is at 1 am in the morning. Since her bathroom is outside of the house she complains that she has to leave the front door open and this is not safe and interrupts her sleep. Maxwell is often left unsupervised in the home and Ms. Wallis leaves his breakfast and lunch for him. He does not go outside and stays in the house until she returns at 5 pm. Maxwell has a new habit of rubbing feces all of the wall of the house and Ms. Wallis thinks this has to do with his medication. He is currently taking Haloperidol and Cholorpromazine among other medications. Ms. Wallis appears frustrated because her house is dilapidated and smells of urine because of her son.

Questions

1. Who is the client?
2. What is the presenting problem?
3. What casework approach would you use for this case and why?
4. Create three questions you would use during the interview.

Janice

Janice is a 35 year old, an African women who is currently working at a bank as a loan officer in Tobago and was referred by the Human Resources Department for employee assistance and counselling. She is 4 ft. 11′ and slightly obese. She appears well groomed and wears a wig. She attend the Anglican Church regularly but does not have a strong spiritual relationship, according to her she does it for appearances only. She is single and has no children.

Janice was born and raised in East Trinidad for Orville and Alice Knightbridge. Orville was a bus driver and Alice was a teacher. She also has two brothers Jeffrey (38) and Jamal (30) and a sister Jacqueline (21) who currently lives in England with an aunt. Janice's parents passed away 5 years ago but was close to Jamal, who she often confides in but he has not been supportive of her during this turbulent period.

Janice attended Eastern Girls College and Arima Anglican School. At the age of 12, Janice was raped by her paternal uncle Jack numerous times and when she complained to her mother about the situation. Her mother hushed her and told her not to repeat the incident. Janice then confided in a close friend Rachel who was older than her about her hate and disgust for men. Rachel held her close for about an hour and told her it was okay to cry and feel the way she was feeling. She explained men are really dirty creatures and Janice should not trust them. After a few months Janice began to have deep feelings for Rachel and they began to have an intimate relationship. Her parents soon found out and her father kicked her out the house and she went to live in Moriah, Tobago with a family friend. Janice continued her education and obtained her six O levels. She also began a relationship with another woman for about 2 years.

Janice obtained a job at the bank and lives on her own. Her family became aware of her sexual orientation and began to distance themselves from her. Even her brother Jamal is no longer available to talk to her like he used too. Janice started a new relationship with Sherry, who is a police officer. They bought a house and they live together. Sherry began to physically abut Janice because of her drinking. Janice is presently drinking up to four drinks a night. Janice met Sherry at a party and they started dating each other for the last 4 years. Sherry was very protective of Janice and was very kind to her. They share the bills in the home and take trips around the Caribbean. About 1 year ago, Sherry commented that she noticed Janice was drinking too much and too often. Janice did not see it as a problem and continued drinking. One night Janice and Sherry were at a party and Janice passed out on the floor. Sherry was so embarrassed that when they arrived home Sherry slapped Janice and told her to stop drinking. Janice complied for a couple of months and returned to drinking again. Ever since Sherry has been hitting her at least once a week. They have stopped sleeping together and now Janice sleeps on the couch.

Janice is experience difficulty functioning at work and grieves tearfully for the loss of her both parents, although she was kicked out of her home at an early age. Janice also complains about the lack of communication with her siblings and aunts and uncles.

Questions

1. What is the presenting problem?
2. What casework approach would you use for this case and why?
3. Create three questions you would use during the interview.

Alicia

Alicia is an 11 year old female who was referred to the Child Guidance Clinic from the San Juan Health facility due to her exhibiting abnormal behavior towards her siblings and peers at school.

Alicia's father was deported from Canada when he was 23 years old because he was allegedly involved with selling illegal drugs. Upon his return to Trinidad, he resided with his grandmother. Alicia's father Joseph met her mother Erin when she was 17 years old. They shared a visiting relationship because Joseph's grandmother did not approve of the relationship. However, Erin would stay with Joseph at his home unbeknownst to his grandmother. Other times Erin lived with her mother. A year into the on-again off again relationship Erin became pregnant with Alicia. After her birth Erin began to use marijuana and (pipe) cocaine with Joseph. Their union produced four children Alicia (11), Jarad (10), Simone (8) and Afia (13 months). Joseph seldom worked construction and was supported by his grandmother. It is alleged that the couple would take the children to the mall to shoplift and beg.

When Alicia was 8 years old her younger sister Afia died at 13 months old. Afia's death was under investigation because of some bruising on her body. The autopsy revealed that cause of death was pneumonia and bruising caused by administration of CPR. About a year after Afia's death, Erin ended the relationship stating she was tired of the drug use, Joseph's possessiveness and his physical and sexual abuse.

On March 2011, Erin's mother filed for legal custody of the children and was granted care and control of the children. She shared custody with the biological parents who were allowed liberal access. Also in 2011 Erin began another relationship with another young gentleman Joey, moved in with Joey and left the children in the care of her mother. Erin and Joey lived together for 2 years but Joseph wanted to reconcile with Erin and she did not. According to Erin, Joseph would stalk her and threatened to burn down the place where she was staying. Erin ended the relationship when Joseph was arrested and charged with a drug offense. At that time Erin and Joseph briefly reconciled.

By the end of 2011, Joseph was enrolled in the drug rehabilitation programme at the New Life Ministries Drug Rehabilitation Centre at Mt. St. Benedict. Erin never entered a drug rehabilitation program while Joseph finished one program and entered into the Piparo Empowerment Centre. However he left the program 1 month earlier and was living with his children and Erin's mother. Erin's mother stated they attended church regularly and Joseph would take the children to visit with his grandmother on Sundays.

In early 2012, Erin entered another relationship with a fellow named Sebastian. Sabastian was both a friend of Erin's and Joseph's. On September 2012 at 5 p.m. Erin's mother called for Joseph to bring the children home as they were visiting his grandmother. Alicia called her mother to come over to help her with a school project. Joseph put his son Jarad to bed as he had a stomach ache. It is alleged upon the arrival of Erin and Sabastian an argument between Joseph and Sabastian ensued. Joseph asked Erin to tell Sabastian to leave. Erin and Sabastian left the house and Joseph followed them out of the house. Sabastian refused to leave and was leaning against his car speaking with a neighbour. Erin saw Sabastian pull something out his care and push Joseph, a scuffle ensued. Sabastian and Joseph fought for a little while and then Joseph fell to the ground. Erin's mother saw Sabastian with a bloody pen knife in his hand. Joseph got up and walked around the front yard saying Erin looked what you caused and then collapsed and died.

Sabastian was held that night by police at Four Roads police station but was later on freed on self- defense.

As Alicia witnessed the entire incident her behavior has changed. Her mother still lives with Sabastian. Alicia becomes very sensitive towards topics regarding her mother. Alicia will slap and cuff her younger siblings. Alicia stated that if Erin her mother becomes pregnant by Sabastian she will kill the baby. Alicia also does not want to attend school.

Questions

1. What is the presenting problem?
2. What casework approach would you use for this case and why?
3. Create three questions you would use during the interview.

Laure

Laure is a 61 year old, an African Trinidadian male who was referred to the Mt. Hope Medical Clinic social work department because of moles on his penis that hurt when he is having sexual intercouse. Laure is a clean, neatly dressed genetleman with a polo shirt tucked into his pants. He has a recently shaved beard and a low haircut. He is calm and he maintained good eye contact.

Laure was the first of two boys born to Mavis Smalls and Darwin Padels. As parents they had an on again, off again common-in-law relationship until his father left when Laure was 6 years old. Laure never saw his father again and his mother took care of him and his bother on her own. Laure recalls at age twelve he heard his father was killed in an altercation with another man. He was 43 years old at the time. His mother cleaned homes and washed clothes for a living. Laure remember fondly that she was hardworking and made sure they were clean and had food to eat. Mavis had another relationship some years afterwards with another man name Charles, they eventually married after 3 years. Laure was about 10 years old.

Laure attended a primary school in Port-of-Spain until he was in fifth standard level. Laure learned a trade in construction where he worked for many years.

Laure remembered after his mother got married, they as a family attended the Seventh-day Adventist services regularly. It was around that time the entire family were baptized and things changed for the better. Laure felt Charles treated he and his brother like his own children and he was very good to his mother. Laure's mother passed 4 years ago at the age of 83. Laure admits at the time of his mother's death he was in a depressed mood occasionally.

Laure went to live on his own at 28 years old and during that time he confessed his church attendance declined and he started smoking cigarettes and drinking alcohol. Laure stated he stopped smoking 10 years ago but continues to drink alcohol socially with friends. Laure however, maintains he still prays and reads the bible.

Laure was never married but fathered two children Junior 32 years old and Abbey 29 years old during a common-in-law relationship with Joan which ended 4 years after the birth of his second child Abbey. His daughter Abbey lives in Tobago and is married and his son junior is very supportive of him and sees him regularly. Since then Luare has not maintained a stable relationship for the past 20 years. He considers his sexual activity is sporadic and when he does have sexual relations he uses a condom at times but asserts that his sexual partners are people he 'knew' for some time. Luare admitted to have gonococcal infection more than a year ago but failed to seek help for it and opted to treat it himself. Since then he has had no problems until 'moles' appeared on his penis. Prior to this visit he has never done a HIV exam and did not know his status. During this visit Laure has been told that he is indeed HIV positive.

Questions

1. What is the presenting problem?
2. What casework approach would you use for this case and why?
3. Create three questions you would use during the interview.

Janice

Janice is a 35 year old, an African women who is currently working at a bank as a loan officer in Tobago and was referred by the Human Resources Department for employee assistance and counselling. She is 4 ft. 11′ and slightly obese. She appears well groomed and wears a wig. She attend the Anglican Church regularly but does not have a strong spiritual relationship, according to her she does it for appearances only. She is single and has no children.

Janice was born and raised in East Trinidad for Orville and Alice Knightbridge. Orville was a bus driver and Alice was a teacher. She also has two brothers Jeffrey (38) and Jamal (30) and a sister Jacqueline (21) who currently lives in England with an aunt. Janice's parents passed away 5 years ago but was close to Jamal, who she often confides in but he has not been supportive of her during this turbulent period.

Janice attended Eastern Girls College and Arima Anglican School. At the age of 12, Janice was raped by her paternal uncle Jack numerous times and when she complained to her mother about the situation. Her mother hushed her and told her not to repeat the incident. Janice then confided in a close friend Rachel who was older than her about her hate and disgust for men. Rachel held her close for about an hour and told her it was okay to cry and feel the way she was feeling. She explained men are really dirty creatures and Janice should not trust them. After a few months Janice began to have deep feelings for Rachel and they began to have an intimate relationship. Her parents soon found out and her father kicked her out the house and she went to live in Moriah, Tobago with a family friend. Janice continued her education and obtained her six O levels. She also began a relationship with another woman for about 2 years.

Janice obtained a job at the bank and lives on her own. Her family became aware of her sexual orientation and began to distance themselves from her. Even her brother Jamal is no longer available to talk to her like he used too. Janice started a new relationship with Sherry, who is a police officer. They bought a house and they live together. Sherry began to physically abut Janice because of her drinking. Janice is presently drinking up to four drinks a night. Janice met Sherry at a party and they started dating each other for the last 4 years. Sherry was very protective of Janice and was very kind to her. They share the bills in the home and take trips around the Caribbean. About 1 year ago, Sherry commented that she noticed Janice was drinking too much and too often. Janice did not see it as a problem and continued drinking. One night Janice and Sherry were at a party and Janice passed out on the floor. Sherry was so embarrassed that when they arrived home Sherry slapped Janice and told her to stop drinking. Janice complied for a couple of months and returned to drinking again. Ever since Sherry has been hitting her at least once a week. They have stopped sleeping together and now Janice sleeps on the couch.

Janice is experience difficulty functioning at work and grieves tearfully for the loss of her both parents, although she was kicked out of her home at an early age. Janice also complains about the lack of communication with her siblings and aunts and uncles.

Questions

1. What is the presenting problem?
2. What casework approach would you use for this case and why?
3. Create three questions you would use during the interview.

References

American Psychiatric Association. (2013). *Diagnostic an statistical manual of mental disorders* (5th ed.). Washington, DC: Author.

Compton, B., & Galaway, B. (Eds.). (1994). *Social work process* (5th ed.). Pacific Grove: Brooks/Cole.

Gerlfand, B. (1988). *The creative practitioner: Creative theory and method for the helping services*. New York: Haworth Press.

Johnson, E. J. (2018). A case study on the consequences of HIV/AIDS within the Caribbean: Issues faced by a teenager born with HIV: *HIV & AIDS Review. International Journal of HIV related problems*

Mayer, R. (1994). Problem solving. In *Encyclopaedia of human behavior* (Vol. 3, pp. 599–602). San Diego: Academic.

Osmo, R., & Rosen, A. (1994). Problem specificity and use of problem solving strategies. *Journal of Social Service Research, 20*, 1/2.

Perlman, H. (1957). *Social casework: A problem-solving process*. Chicago: University of Chicago Press.

Reid, W. (1996). Task-centered social work. In F. Turner (Ed.), *Social work treatment: Interlocking theoretical approaches* (4th ed., pp. 617–640). New York: Free Press.

Thomlison, B., & Thomlison, R. (1996). Behavior theory and social work treatment. In F. Turner (Ed.), *Social work treatment: Interlocking theoretical approaches* (4th ed., pp. 39–68). New York: Free Press.

Turner, F., & Jaco, R. M. (1996). Problem-solving theory and social work treatment. In F. Turner (Ed.), *Social work treatment: Interlocking theoretical approaches* (4th ed., pp. 503–522). New York: Free Press.

Index

E. J. Johnson, C. L. Huggins, *Social Casework Methodology: A Skills Handbook for the Caribbean Human Services Worker*, SpringerBriefs in Social Work,
https://doi.org/10.1007/978-3-030-27319-4